Pocket Guide to
NURSING DIAGNOSES

Pocket Guide to NURSING DIAGNOSES

Edited by

MI JA KIM, R.N., Ph.D., F.A.A.N.
Associate Professor, College of Nursing,
University of Illinois at Chicago,
Health Sciences Center,
Chicago, Illinois

GERTRUDE K. McFARLAND, R.N., D.N.Sc.
Nurse Consultant, Division of Nursing,
USPHS, Health Resources and Services Administration,
U.S. Department of Health and Human Services,
Rockville, Maryland

AUDREY M. McLANE, R.N., Ph.D.
Professor, College of Nursing,
Marquette University,
Milwaukee, Wisconsin

The C. V. Mosby Company

ST. LOUIS   TORONTO   1984

MOSBY

A TRADITION OF PUBLISHING EXCELLENCE

Editor: Barbara Ellen Norwitz
Assistant editor: Sally Adkisson
Manuscript editor: Lois Brunngraber
Design: Jeanne E. Genz
Production: Barbara Merritt, Teresa Breckwoldt

Printed in the United States of America

The C.V. Mosby Company
11830 Westline Industrial Drive, St. Louis, Missouri 63146

Library of Congress Cataloging in Publication Data
Main entry under title:

Pocket guide to nursing diagnoses.

  1. Diagnosis.   2. Nursing.   I. Kim, Mi Ja.
II. McFarland, Gertrude K.   III. McLane,
Audrey M.   [DNLM: 1. Nursing process.   2. Patient
care planning.   WY 100 P739]
RT48.P63   1984   616.07′5   83-23632
ISBN   0-8016-2672-2

GW/D/D   9   8   7   6   5   4   3   03/A/324

CONTRIBUTORS

LUCY FEILD, R.N., M.S.N.
Brigham and Women's Hospital, Boston, Massachusetts

PAMELA GOTCH, R.N., M.S.N.
Marquette University, Milwaukee, Wisconsin

MEG GULANICK, R.N., M.S.N.
Michael Reese Hospital, Chicago, Illinois; University of Illinois at Chicago, Health Sciences Center, Chicago, Illinois

DOROTHEA F. JAKOB, R.N., M.A.
Department of Public Health, Toronto, Canada

MI JA KIM, R.N., Ph.D., F.A.A.N.
University of Illinois at Chicago, Health Sciences Center, Chicago, Illinois

DONNA LAWRENCE, R.N., M.S.N.
Marquette University, Milwaukee, Wisconsin

GERTRUDE K. McFARLAND, R.N., D.N.Sc.*
Division of Nursing, USPHS, Health Resources and Services Administration, U.S. Department of Health and Human Services, Rockville, Maryland

AUDREY M. McLANE, R.N., Ph.D.
Marquette University, Milwaukee, Wisconsin

JACQUELINE MILLER, R.N., M.S.
Department of Health and Social Services, Madison, Wisconsin

---

*The opinions expressed herein are those of the authors and do not necessarily reflect those of the U.S. Department of Health and Human Services, USPHS, Health Resources and Services Administration.

MARGARET J. STAFFORD, R.N., M.S.N., F.A.A.N.
Hines Veterans Administration Hospital, Hines, Illinois;
University of Illinois at Chicago, Health Sciences Center,
Chicago, Ilinois

KATHLYN STEELE, R.N., M.S.
Department of Health and Social Services, Madison,
Wisconsin

EVELYN L. WASLI, R.N., M.S.N., D.N.Sc.*
St. Elizabeths Hospital, National Institute of Mental
Health, U.S. Public Health Service, U.S. Department
of Health and Human Services, Washington, D.C.

---

*The opinions expressed herein are those of the authors and do
not necessarily reflect those of St. Elizabeths Hospital or the
National Institute of Mental Health.

CONTENTS

INTRODUCTION

This pocket guide of nursing diagnoses is organized in three sections. The first section includes definitions of a nursing diagnosis and guidelines for preparing a diagnostic category, the second includes a list of approved nursing diagnoses, and the third provides some prototype care plans incorporating nursing diagnoses.

In the first section the authors aim to establish a baseline for common understanding of nursing diagnosis among the users of this manual. Representative definitions of nursing diagnosis are offered by M. Gordon (1976), C. Roy (1982), and J. Shoemaker (1984).

The second section presents all nursing diagnoses that were approved at the Fifth National Conference on Classification of Nursing Diagnosis held in St. Louis, Missouri, in April 1982. No new diagnoses were approved at the Sixth National Conference in 1984; therefore the book contains the most current information available on nursing diagnoses. It reflects the refinement of the nursing diagnosis from the Fourth National Conference and includes eight new diagnoses. There were numerous new defining characteristics suggested at the Fifth National Conference for existing nursing diagnoses, and these are identified with † marks. Defining characteristics that small groups suggested for deletion were omitted from the list but included in the comment section under each nursing diagnosis. However, it should be kept in mind that the Task Force of the National Group for the Classification of Nursing Diagnoses did not have sufficient time to scrutinize these characteristics and ap-

---

* See end of Section I for all references.

prove them individually. Therefore, the characteristics have not been formally approved by the National Conference group. The nursing diagnoses are presented alphabetically for ready use by professional nurses in their practice. A listing of the diagnostic labels accepted at the Third National Conference (which updated the First and Second National Conference) is added to this section to present a historic perspective of the diagnostic labels. Etiologies and defining characteristics associated with the listings of the Third National Conference can be found in the Proceedings of the Third and Fourth National Conference (Kim and Moritz, 1982*).

The third section illustrates how nursing diagnoses can be incorporated into the problem-solving process in nursing practice. This section was designed by the editors of the Proceedings with the thought that some examples of the use of nursing diagnoses in practice would facilitate the understanding and the use of nursing diagnoses. Care plans were developed by experts in respective specialty areas from different parts of the nation, and we recognize the limited coverage of the specialty areas. The editors wish to acknowledge that the materials contained in this section were solicited after the conference and reflect the opinions of the individual authors and not necessarily those of the North American Nursing Diagnosis Association.

Readers of the manual are referred to the main text. *Classification of Nursing Diagnoses: Proceedings of the Fifth National Conference* (Kim et al., 1984*), for comprehensive coverage of the subject matter, nursing diagnosis. Nurses who gain expertise from the use of these nursing diagnoses are urged to share their data and insights at local, regional, and national conferences. Through such mechanisms all nurses can participate in the generation of knowledge for nursing science.

---

* See end of Section I for all references.

Definition of nursing diagnosis and guidelines for preparing diagnostic categories

Definitions of Nursing Diagnosis

"Nursing diagnosis made by professional nurses describes actual or potential health problems that nurses, by virtue of their education and experience, are capable and licensed to treat" (Gordon, 1976, p. 1299).

Nursing diagnosis is a concise phrase or term summarizing a cluster of empirical indicators representing patterns of unitary man (Roy, 1982).

"A nursing diagnosis is a clinical judgment about an individual, family, or community which is derived through a deliberate, systematic process of data collection and analysis. It provides the basis for prescriptions for definitive therapy for which the nurse is accountable. It is expressed concisely and it includes the etiology of the condition when known" (Shoemaker, 1984, p. 94).

Guidelines for Preparing Diagnostic Categories (Gordon, 1982)

In making a nursing diagnosis, a nurse places a patient (client) in a diagnostic category for purposes of determining therapy. Diagnostic categories can be at different levels of abstraction. Those that are clinically useful are sufficiently specific to permit determination of a plan of therapy. For example, if nursing is concerned with human functions and their alterations, a broad category of problems and potential problems would be Alterations in Bowel Elimination. At the next level of abstraction there might be Deficiencies and Excesses. *Usually* found at the next level are the clinically useful diagnoses, for example, constipation, diarrhea, and so forth. Category levels should describe health problems at a clinically useful level of abstraction.

A diagnostic category has three parts: (1) the term(s) describing the problem or the category label (P); (2) the probable cause of the problem, the etiologic subcategory (E); and (3) the defining characteristics, the signs and symptoms (S). The following are characteristics of each part of a diagnostic category:

A. The category label (or title)
   1. The label is a term(s) that describes a client (individual, family, community) health problem.
   2. The label refers to an identifiable clinical entity (health problem) that nurses can identify and treat.
   3. The label is clear and concise.
   4. The label is sufficiently specific to be clinically useful.
B. Common etiologic factors: the etiologic subcategory (if it can be identified)
   1. An etiologic subcategory is a term(s) describing one (or more) probable cause(s) of the health problem.
   2. The etiologic subcategory when combined with the category label suggests a treatment plan.
   3. The terms describing the etiologic subcategory are clear and concise.
   4. The terms describing the etiologic subcategory are sufficiently specific to be clinically useful.
C. The defining characteristics of the diagnostic category
   1. The defining characteristics are *observable* signs and symptoms that are present when the health problem is present or when the diagnostic category is used clinically.

REFERENCES

Gordon, M.: Nursing diagnosis and the diagnostic process, Am. J. Nurs. 76:1298-1300, 1976.

Gordon, M.: Guidelines for reviewing and preparing diagnostic categories. In Kim, M.J., and Moritz, D.A., editors: Classification of nursing diagnoses: proceedings of the Third and Fourth National Conferences, New York, 1982, McGraw-Hill Book Co.

Kim, M.J., McFarland, G.K., and McLane, A.M., editors: Classifications of nursing diagnoses: proceedings of the Fifth National Conference, St. Louis, 1984, The C.V. Mosby Co.

Kim, M.J., and Moritz, D.A., editors: Classification of nursing diagnoses: proceedings of the Third and Fourth National Conferences, New York, 1982, McGraw-Hill Book Co., pp. 321-338.

Roy, C.: Theoretical framework for classification of nursing diagnosis. In Kim, M.J., and Moritz, D.A., editors: Classification of nursing diagnoses: proceedings of the Third and Fourth National Conferences, New York, 1982, McGraw-Hill Book Co.

Shoemaker, J.: Essential features of nursing diagnosis. In Kim, M.J., McFarland, G.K., and McLane, A.M., editors: Classification of nursing diagnoses: proceedings of the Fifth National Conference, St. Louis, 1984, The C.V. Mosby Co.

List of approved nursing diagnoses with etiology and defining characteristics

Activity Intolerance

Etiology
    Generalized weakness
    Sedentary life-style
    Imbalance between oxygen supply and demand
    Bed rest or immobility
Defining characteristics
    *Verbal report of fatigue or weakness
    Abnormal heart rate or blood pressure response to activity
    Exertional discomfort or dyspnea
    Electrocardiographic changes reflecting arrhythmias or ischemia

COMMENT: New diagnosis

Activity Intolerance, Potential

Etiology
    To be developed
Defining characteristics
    History of previous intolerance
    Deconditioned status
    Presence of circulatory/respiratory problems
    Inexperience with the activity

Airway Clearance, Ineffective

Etiology
    Decreased energy and fatigue
    Tracheobronchial
        Infection
        Obstruction
        Secretion
    Perceptual/cognitive impairment
    Trauma

Throughout this section * indicates a critical defining characteristic and † indicates an addition suggested at Fifth National Conference.

Defining characteristics

Abnormal breath sounds—rales (crackles), rhonchi (wheezes)

Changes in rate or depth of respiration

Tachypnea

Cough, effective or ineffective; with or without sputum

Cyanosis

Dyspnea

†Fever

Anxiety

Definition: A vague uneasy feeling, the source of which is often nonspecific or unknown to the individual.

Etiology

Unconscious conflict about essential values and goals of life

Threat to self-concept

Threat of death

Threat to or change in health status

Threat to or change in socioeconomic status

Threat to or change in role functioning

Threat to or change in environment

Threat to or change in interaction patterns

Situational & maturational crises

Interpersonal transmission & contagion

Unmet needs

Defining characteristics

Subjective

Increased tension

Apprehension

Increased helplessness

Uncertainty

Fearful

Scared

Feelings of inadequacy

Shakiness

Fear of unspecific consequences

Regretful
Overexcited
Rattled
Distressed
Jittery
Objective
    *Sympathetic stimulation—cardiovascular excitation, superficial vasoconstriction, pupil dilation
Restlessness
Insomnia
Glancing about
Poor eye contact
Trembling; hand tremors
Extraneous movements—foot shuffling; hand, arm movements
Expressed concern regarding changes in life events
Worried
Anxious
Facial tension
Voice quivering
Focus on self
Increased wariness
Increased perspiration

COMMENTS: New diagnosis

Bowel Elimination, Alteration in: Constipation

Etiology
   †Less than adequate intake
   †Less than adequate dietary intake and bulk
   †Less than adequate physical activity or immobility
   †Personal habits
   †Medications
   †Chronic use of medication and enemas
   †Gastrointestinal obstructive lesions
   †Neuromuscular impairment

†Musculoskeletal impairment
†Pain on defecation
†Diagnostic procedures
†Lack of privacy
†Weak abdominal musculature
†Pregnancy
†Emotional status

Defining characteristics
Frequency less than usual pattern
Hard-formed stool
Palpable mass
Reported feeling of rectal fullness
Straining at stool
†Decreased bowel sounds
†Reported feeling of abdominal or rectal fullness or pressure
†Less than usual amount of stool
†Nausea

Other possible defining characteristics
Abdominal pain
Back pain
Headache
Interference with daily living
Use of laxatives
†Decreased appetite
Appetite impairment

COMMENTS: The following defining characteristics were deleted: decreased activity level; reported feeling of pressure in rectum; and appetite impairment.

Bowel Elimination, Alteration in: Diarrhea

Etiology
†Stress & anxiety
†Dietary intake
†Medications
†Inflammation, irritation, or malabsorption of bowel

†Toxins
†Contaminants
†Radiation
Defining characteristics
Abdominal pain
Cramping
Increased frequency
Increased frequency of bowel sounds
Loose, liquid stools
Urgency
†Changes in color

Bowel Elimination, Alteration in: Incontinence

Etiology
†Neuromuscular involvement
†Musculoskeletal involvement
†Depression; severe anxiety
†Perception or cognitive impairment
Defining characteristics
*Involuntary passage of stool

COMMENTS: More specific signs and symptoms are still needed.

Breathing Pattern, Ineffective

Etiology
Neuromuscular impairment
Pain
Musculoskeletal impairment
Perception or cognitive impairment
Anxiety
Decreased energy and fatigue
†Inflammatory process
†Decreased lung expansion
†Tracheobronchial obstruction

Defining characteriestics
    Dyspnea
    Shortness of breath
    Tachypnea
    Fremitus
    Abnormal arterial blood gas
    Cyanosis
    Cough
    Nasal flaring
    Respiratory depth changes
    Assumption of 3-point position
    Pursed-lip breathing and prolonged expiratory phase
    Increased anteroposterior diameter
    Use of accessory muscles
    Altered chest excursion

Cardiac Output, Alteration in: Decreased

Etiology
    Mechanical
        †Alteration in preload
        †Alteration in afterload
        †Alteration in inotropic changes in heart
    Electrical
        †Alterations in rate
        †Alterations in rhythm
        †Alteration in conduction
    Structural
Defining characteristics
    †Variations in hemodynamic readings
    Arrhythmias; ECG changes
    Fatigue
    Jugular vein distension
    †Cyanosis; pallor of skin and mucous membranes
    †Oliguria; anuria
    Decreased peripheral pulses
    Cold, clammy skin
    Rales
    Dyspnea

Orthopnea
Restlessness
Other possible defining characteristics
Change in mental status
Shortness of breath
Syncope
Vertigo
Edema
Cough
Frothy sputum
Gallop rhythm; abnormal heart sounds
Weakness

COMMENTS: Further development of this diagnosis in the framework of nursing practice is recommended. Debate continues whether this problem can be independently treated by nurses or whether it falls more into the collaborative realm. Some felt "other possible defining characteristics" should be deleted. The following defining characteristics were modified: variations in blood pressure readings; and color changes, skin and mucous membranes. Suggested changes and additions are viewed as extension of existing defining characteristics, hence no research data are required to support them.

Comfort, Alteration in: Pain

Etiology
Injuring agents
Biologic
Chemical
Physical
Psychologic
Defining characteristics
Subjective
Communication (verbal or coded) of pain descriptors

Objective

Guarding behavior; protective

Self-focusing

Narrowed focus (altered time perception, withdrawal from social contact, impaired thought process)

Distraction behavior (moaning, crying, pacing, seeking out other people and/or activities, restlessness)

Facial mask of pain (eyes lack luster, "beaten look," fixed or scattered movement, grimace)

Alteration in muscle tone (may span from listless to rigid)

Autonomic responses not seen in chronic, stable pain (diaphoresis, blood pressure and pulse rate change, pupillary dilation, increased or decreased respiratory rate)

Communication, Impaired: Verbal

Etiology [1]

Decrease in circulation to the brain

Physical barrier, brain tumor, tracheostomy, intubation

Anatomic deficit, cleft palate

Psychologic barriers, psychosis, lack of stimuli

Cultural difference

Developmental or age-related

Defining characteristics

*Unable to speak dominant language

*Does not or cannot speak

Stuttering; slurring

---

[1] Different organization of etiology suggested at Fifth National Conference is listed under Issue section of the same diagnosis in Kim, M. J., McLane, A. M., and McFarland, G. K., editors: Classification of nursing diagnosis: proceedings of the Fifth National Conference, St. Louis, 1984, The C. V. Mosby Co.

†Impaired articulation
Dyspnea
Disorientation
†Inability to modulate speech
†Inability to find words
†Inability to name words
†Inability to identify objects
†Loose association of ideas
†Flight of ideas
†Incessant verbalization
†Difficulty with phonation
†Inability to speak in sentences

COMMENTS: Following defining characteristics were deleted: speaks or verbalizes with difficulty; difficulty forming words or sentences; difficulty expressing thought verbally; and inappropriate verbalization.

Coping, Family: Potential for Growth

Definition: The family member has effectively managed adaptive tasks involved with the client's health challenge and is exhibiting desire and readiness for enhanced health and growth in regard to self and in relation to the client.

Etiology

The person's basic needs are sufficiently gratified and adaptive tasks effectively addressed to enable goals of self-actualization to surface.

Defining characteristics

Family members attempt to describe growth impact of crisis on their own values, priorities, goals, or relationships.

Family member is moving in direction of health-promoting and enriching life-style that supports and monitors maturational processes, audits and negotiates treatment programs, and generally chooses experiences that optimize wellness.

Individual expresses interest in making contact on a one-to-one basis or on a mutual-aid group basis with another person who has experienced a similar situation.

COMMENT: Degree of independent nursing therapy: high.

Coping, Ineffective Family: Compromised

Definition: A usually supportive primary person (family member or close friend) is providing insufficient, ineffective, or compromised support, comfort, assistance, or encouragement that may be needed by the client to manage or master adaptive tasks related to the client's health challenge.

Etiology

Inadequate or incorrect information or understanding by a primary person

Temporary preoccupation by a significant person who is trying to manage emotional conflicts and personal suffering and is unable to perceive or act effectively in regard to client's needs

Temporary family disorganization and role changes

Other situational or developmental crises or situations the significant person may be facing

Client providing little support in turn for the primary person

Prolonged disease or disability progression that exhausts the supportive capacity of significant people

Defining characteristics

Subjective

Client expresses or confirms a concern or complaint about significant other's response to client's health problem

Significant person describes preoccupation with personal reactions, e.g., fear, anticipatory grief, guilt, anxiety regarding client's illness or disability, or to other situational or developmental crises

Significant person describes or confirms an inadequate understanding or knowledge base that interferes with effective assistive or supportive behaviors

Objective

Significant person attempts assistive or supportive behaviors with less than satisfactory results

Significant person withdraws or enters into limited or temporary personal communication with client at time of need

Significant person displays protective behavior disproportionate (too little or too much) to client's abilities or need for autonomy

COMMENTS: Degree of independent nursing therapy: high. Differential diagnosing: the coping strategies of family members addressed in this diagnosis are basically constructive in nature. The constructive but compromised response and intent fall short of their realistic potential for effective situation or crisis management.

Coping, Ineffective Family: Disabling

Definition: The behavior of a significant person (family member or other primary person) disables his or her own capacities and the client's capacities to effectively address tasks essential to either person's adaptation to the health challenge.

Etiology

Significant person with chronically unexpressed feelings of guilt, anxiety, hostility, despair, etc.

Dissonant discrepancy of coping styles being used to deal with the adaptive tasks by the significant person and client or among significant people

Highly ambivalent family relationships

Arbitrary handling of a family's resistance to treatment which tends to solidify defensiveness as it fails to deal adequately with underlying anxiety

Defining characteristics

Neglectful care of the client in regard to basic human needs and/or illness treatment

Distortion of reality regarding the client's health problem, including extreme denial about its existence or severity

Intolerance

Rejection

Abandonment

Desertion

Carrying on usual routines; disregarding client's needs

Psychosomatic tendency

Taking on illness signs of client

Decisions and actions by family which are detrimental to economic or social well-being

Agitation, depression, aggression, hostility

Impaired restructuring of a meaningful life for self; impaired individualization; prolonged overconcern for client

Neglectful relationships with other family members

Client's development of helpless, inactive dependence

COMMENTS: Degree of independent nursing therapy: moderate to high. Regarding the family member's disabling coping response to the client's health challenge, one can describe a family member's response as disabling if it involves short-term coping behaviors that are highly detrimental to the welfare of the client or the significant person. In addition, chronically disabling patterns by a primary person are described as continued use of selected coping skills that have interrupted the person's longer-term capacity to receive, store, or organize information or to react to it.

Coping, Ineffective Individual

Definition: Ineffective coping is the impairment of adaptive behaviors and problem-solving abilities of a person in meeting life's demands and roles.

19

Etiology
  Situation crises
  Maturational crises
  Personal vulnerability
  †Multiple life changes
  †No vacations
  †Inadequate relaxation
  †Inadequate support systems
  †Little or no exercise
  †Poor nutrition
  †Unmet expectations
  †Work overload
  †Too many deadlines
  †Unrealistic perceptions
  †Inadequate coping method
Defining Characteristics
  *Verbalization of inability to cope or inability to ask
    for help
  Inability to meet role expectations
  Inability to meet basic needs
  *Inability to problem-solve
  Alteration in societal participation
  Destructive behavior toward self or others
  Inappropriate use of defense mechanisms
  Change in usual communication patterns
  Verbal manipulation
  High illness rate
  High rate of accidents
  †Overeating
  †Lack of appetite
  †Excessive smoking
  †Excessive drinking
  †Overuse of prescribed tranquilizers
  †Alcohol proneness
  †High blood pressure
  †Chronic fatigue
  †Insomnia
  †Muscular tension

20

†Ulcers
†Frequent headaches
†Frequent neckaches
†Irritable bowel
†Chronic worry
†General irritability
†Poor self-esteem
†Chronic anxiety
†Emotional tension
†Chronic depression

Diversional Activity, Deficit

Etiology
Environmental lack of diversional activity
Long-term hospitalization
Frequent, lengthy treatments
Defining characteristics
Patient's statement regarding the following:
Boredom
Wish there were something to do, to read, etc.
Usual hobbies cannot be undertaken in hospital

Family Process, Alteration in

Etiology
Situation transition and/or crises
Development transition and/or crises
Defining characteristics[1]
Family system unable to meet physical needs for its
members
Family system unable to meet emotional needs of its
members

---

[1] The first 13 defining characteristics are specifically from Otto,
H.: Criteria for assessing family strengths, Fam. Process 2:329-
338, Sept. 1963.

21

Family system unable to meet spiritual needs of its members

Parents do not demonstrate respect for each other's views on child-rearing practices

Inability to express or accept wide range of feelings

Inability to express or accept feelings of members

Family unable to meet security needs of its members

Inability of family members to relate to each other for mutual growth and maturation

Family uninvolved in community activities

Inability to accept or receive help appropriately

Rigidity in function and roles

Family does not demonstrate respect for individuality and autonomy of its members

Family inability to adapt to change or to deal with traumatic experience constructively

Family fails to accomplish current or past developmental task

Ineffective family decision-making process

Failure to send and receive clear messages

Inappropriate boundary maintenance

Inappropriate or poorly communicated family rules, rituals, symbols

Unexamined family myths

Inappropriate level and direction of energy

COMMENTS: New diagnosis

Fear

Definition: Fear is a feeling of dread related to an identifiable source which the person validates.

†**Etiology**

Natural or innate origins—sudden noise, loss of physical support, height, pain

Learned response—conditioning, modeling from or identification with others

Separation from support system in a potentially threatening situation (hospitalization, treatments, etc.)
Knowledge deficit or unfamiliarity
Language barrier
Sensory impairment
Phobic stimulus or phobia
Environmental stimuli
†**Defining Characteristics**
　Subjective
　　Increased tension
　　Apprehension
　　Impulsiveness
　　Decreased self-assurance
　　Afraid
　　Scared
　　Terrified
　　Panic
　　Frightened
　　Jittery
　Objective
　　Increased alertness
　　Concentration on source
　　Wide-eyed
　　Attack behavior
　　Focus on "it, out there"
　　Fight behavior—aggressive
　　Flight behavior—withdrawal
　　Sympathetic stimulation—cardiovascular excitation, superficial vasoconstriction, pupil dilation

COMMENTS: Previous defining characteristic, ability to identify object of fear (knowing), was deleted. At the Fourth National Conference some group members expressed concern over the fact that fear may be a symptom of ineffective coping with others. As the diagnosis is further developed, it may be discovered that fear is not an appropriate nursing diagnosis and is a symptom analogous to the symptom of anxiety.

Fluid Volume, Alteration in: Excess

Etiology
  Compromised regulatory mechanism
  Excess fluid intake
  Excess sodium intake
Defining characteristics
  Edema
  Effusion
  Anasarca
  Weight gain
  Shortness of breath, orthopnea
  Intake greater than output
  Third heart sound
  Pulmonary congestion on x-ray film
  Abnormal breath sounds: crackles (rales)
  Change in respiratory pattern
  Change in mental status
  Decreased hemoglobin, hematocrit
  Blood pressure changes
  Central venous pressure changes
  Pulmonary artery pressure changes
  Jugular venous distention
  Positive hepatojugular reflex
  Oliguria
  Specific gravity changes
  Azoturia
  Altered electrolytes
  Restlessness and anxiety

COMMENTS: New diagnosis

Fluid Volume Deficit, Actual (1)

Etiology
  Failure of regulatory mechanisms
Defining characteristics
  Dilute urine
  Increased urine output
  Sudden weight loss

Other possible defining characteristics
Possible weight gain
Hypotension
Decreased venous filling
Increased pulse rate
Decreased skin turgor
Decreased pulse volume & pressure
Increased body temperature
Dry skin
Dry mucous membranes
Hemoconcentration
Weakness
Edema
Thirst

Fluid Volume Deficit, Actual (2)

Etiology
Active loss
Defining characteristics
Decreased urine output
Concentrated urine
Output greater than intake
Sudden weight loss
Decreased venous filling
Hemoconcentration
Increased serum sodium
Other possible defining characteristics
Hypotension
Thirst
Increased pulse rate
Decreased skin turgor
Decreased pulse volume & pressure
Change in mental state
Increased body temperature
Dry skin
Dry mucous membranes
Weakness

Fluid Volume Deficit, Potential

Etiology
  Extremes of age
  Extremes of weight
  Excessive losses through normal routes, e.g., diarrhea
  Loss of fluid through abnormal routes, e.g., indwelling
    tubes
  Deviations affecting access to, intake of, or absorption
    of fluids, e.g., physical immobility
  Factors influencing fluid needs, e.g., hypermetabolic
    states
  Knowledge deficiency related to fluid volume
  Medications, e.g., diuretics
Defining characteristics
  Increased fluid output
  Urinary frequency
  Thirst
  Altered intake

COMMENTS: Etiologies listed are high-risk factors that
could lead to the diagnosis.

Gas Exchange, Impaired

Etiology [1]
  Altered oxygen supply
  Alveolar-capillary membrane changes
  Altered blood flow
  Altered oxygen-carrying capacity of blood
Defining characteristics
  Confusion
  Somnolence
  Restlessness
  Irritability
  Inability to move secretions
  Hypercapnea
  Hypoxia

---

[1] Etiology was changed from the following: ventilation, perfusion imbalance.

Grieving, Anticipatory

†Definitions

Anticipatory grieving—grieving before an actual loss

Grief—response to loss

Dysfunctional grieving—delayed or exaggerated response to a perceived actual or potential loss

Etiology

†Perceived potential loss of significant other

†Perceived potential loss of physiopsychosocial well-being

†Perceived potential loss of personal possessions

Defining characteristics

Potential loss of significant object

Expression of distress at potential loss

Denial of potential loss

Guilt

Anger

Sorrow

Choked feelings

Changes in eating habits

Alterations in sleep patterns

Alterations in activity level

Altered libido

Altered communication patterns

Grieving, Dysfunctional

Etiology

Actual or perceived object loss (object loss is used in the broadest sense). Objects include people, possessions, a job, status, home, ideals, parts and processes of the body, etc.

†Thwarted grieving response to a loss

†Absence of anticipatory grieving

†Chronic fatal illness

†Lack of resolution of previous grieving response

†Loss of significant others

†Loss of physiopsychosocial well-being

†Loss of personal possessions

Defining characteristics
  Verbal expression of distress at loss
  Denial of loss
  Expression of guilt
  Expression of unresolved issues
  Anger
  Sadness
  Crying
  Difficulty in expressing loss
  Alterations in
    Eating habits
    Sleep patterns
    Dream patterns
    Activity level
    Libido
  Idealization of lost object
  Reliving of past experiences
  Interference with life functioning
  Developmental regression
  Labile effect
  Alterations in concentration and/or pursuits of tasks

Health Maintenance, Alteration in

Definition: Inability to identify, manage, and/or seek out
  help to maintain health.
Etiology
  Lack of or significant alteration in communication
    skills (written, verbal, and/or gestural)
  Lack of ability to make deliberate and thoughtful judg-
    ments
  Perceptual or cognitive impairment
  Complete or partial lack of gross and/or fine motor
    skills
  Ineffective individual coping; dysfunctional grieving
  Lack of material resource
  Unachieved developmental tasks
  Ineffective family coping: disabling spiritual distress

Defining characteristics

Demonstrated lack of knowledge regarding basic health practices

Demonstrated lack of adaptive behaviors to internal or external environmental changes

Reported or observed inability to take the responsibility for meeting basic health practices in any or all functional pattern areas

History of lack of health-seeking behavior

Expressed interest in improving health behaviors

Reported or observed lack of equipment, financial, and/or other resources

Reported or observed impairment of personal support system

COMMENTS: New diagnosis

Home Maintenance Management, Impaired

Definition: The client is unable to independently maintain a safe, growth-promoting immediate environment.

Etiology

Disease or injury of individual or family member

Insufficient family organization or planning

Insufficient finances

Unfamiliarity with neighborhood resources

Impaired cognitive or emotional functioning

Lack of knowledge

Lack of role modeling

Inadequate support systems

Defining characteristics

Subjective

*Household members express difficulty in maintaining their home in a comfortable fashion

*Household requests assistance with home maintenance

*Household members describe outstanding debts or financial crises

Objective
  Disorderly surroundings
  *Unwashed or unavailable cooking equipment, clothes, or linen
  *Accumulation of dirt, food wastes, or hygienic wastes
  Offensive odors
  Inappropriate household temperature
  *Overtaxed family members, e.g., exhausted, anxious family members
  Lack of necessary equipment or aids
  Presence of vermin or rodents
  *Repeated hygienic disorders, infestations, or infections

Injury: Potential for

Etiology
Interactive conditions between individual and environment which impose a risk to the defensive and adaptive resources of the individual
  Internal factors, host
    Biological
    Chemical
    Physiologic
    Psychologic perception
    Developmental
  External environment
    Biologic
    Chemical
    Physiologic
    Psychologic
    People-provider
Defining characteristics
  Internal
    Biochemical
      Regulatory function
        Sensory dysfunction
        Integrative dysfunction

Effector dysfunction
Tissue hypoxia
Malnutrition
Immune-autoimmune
Abnormal blood profile
    Leukocytosis or leukopenia
    Altered clotting factors
    Thrombocytopenia
    Sickle cell
    Thalassemia
    Decreased hemoglobin
Physical
    Broken skin
    Altered mobility
Developmental
    Age
        Physiologic
        Psychosocial
Psychologic
    Affective
    Orientation
External
    Biologic
        Immunization level of community
        Microorganism
    Chemical
        Pollutants
        Poisons
        Drugs
            Pharmaceutical agents
            Alcohol
            Caffeine
            Nicotine
        Preservatives
        Cosmetics and dyes
        Nutrients (vitamins, food types)
    Physical
        Design, structure, and arrangement of community, building, and/or equipment

Mode of transport/transportation
Nosocomial agents
People-provider
Nosocomial agent
Staffing patterns
Cognitive, affective, and psychomotor factors

Comments: Etiologic factors are interdependent on the epidemiologic model. The outline of characteristics is provided as a framework for future task work; it is not considered to be all-inclusive in nature. Further development is needed. This diagnosis has three subcomponents: A, B, and C.

A. POISONING, POTENTIAL FOR

Definition: The client has accentuated risk of accidental exposure to or ingestion of drugs or dangerous products in doses sufficient to cause poisoning.

Defining characteristics

Internal (individual) factors
    Reduced vision
    Verbalization of occupational setting without adequate safeguards
    Lack of safety or drug education
    Lack of proper precaution
    Cognitive or emotional difficulties
    Insufficient finances
External (environmental) factors
    Large supplies of drugs in house
    Medicines stored in unlocked cabinets accessible to children or confused persons
    Dangerous products placed or stored within the reach of children or confused persons
    Availability of illicit drugs potentially contaminated by poisonous additives
    Flaking, peeling paint or plaster in presence of young children
    Chemical contamination of food and water
    Unprotected contact with heavy metals or chemicals

Paint, lacquer, etc., in poorly ventilated areas or without effective protection

Presence of poisonous vegetation

Presence of atmospheric pollutants

B. SUFFOCATION, POTENTIAL FOR

Definition: The client has accentuated risk of accidental suffocation (inadequate air available for inhalation).

Defining characteristics

Internal (individual) factors[1]

Reduced olfactory sensation

Reduced motor abilities

Lack of safety education

Lack of safety precautions

Cognitive or emotional difficulties

Disease or injury process

External (environmental) factors

Pillow placed in an infant's crib

Vehicle warming in closed garage

Children playing with plastic bags or inserting small objects into their mouths or noses

Discarded or unused refrigerators or freezers without removed doors

Children left unattended in bathtubs or pools

Household gas leaks

Smoking in bed

Use of fuel-burning heaters not vented to outside

Low-strung clothesline

Pacifier hung around infant's head

Eating of large mouthfuls of food

Propped bottle placed in an infant's crib

C. TRAUMA, POTENTIAL FOR

Definition: The client has accentuated risk of accidental tissue injury, e.g., wound, burn, fracture.

---

[1] Consider immunologic incompetence and alterations in reticuloendothelial system.

Defining characteristics

Internal (individual) factors[1]

Weakness

Poor vision

Balancing difficulties

Reduced temperature and/or tactile sensation

Reduced large—or small—muscle coordination

Reduced hand-eye coordination

Lack of safety education

Lack of safety precautions

Insufficient finances to purchase safety equipment or effect repairs

Cognitive or emotional difficulties

History of previous trauma

External (environmental) factors

Slippery floors, e.g., wet or highly waxed

Snow or ice on stairs, walkways

Unanchored rugs

Bathtub without hand grip or antislip equipment

Use of unsteady ladder or chairs

Entering unlighted rooms

Unsturdy or absent stair rails

Unanchored electric wires

Litter or liquid spills on floors or stairways

High beds

Children playing without gates at top of stairs

Obstructed passageways

Unsafe window protection in homes with young children

Inappropriate call-for-aid mechanisms for bed-resting client

Pot handles facing toward front of stove

Bathing in very hot water, e.g., unsupervised bathing of young children

Potential igniting of gas leaks

Delayed lighting of gas burner or oven

Experimenting with chemicals or gasoline

Unscreened fires or heaters

Wearing of plastic aprons or flowing clothing around open flame

Children playing with matches, candles, cigarettes

Inadequately stored combustibles or corrosives, e.g., matches, oily rags, lye

Highly flammable children's toys or clothing

Overloaded fuse boxes

Contact with rapidly moving machinery, industrial belts, or pulleys

Sliding on coarse bed linen or struggling within bed restraints

Faulty electrical plugs, frayed wires, or defective appliances

Contact with acids or alkalis

Playing with fireworks or gunpowder

Contact with intense cold

Overexposure to sun, sun lamps, radiotherapy

Use of cracked dishware or glasses

Knives stored uncovered

Guns or ammunition stored unlocked

Large icicles hanging from roof

Exposure to dangerous machinery

Children playing with sharp-edged toys

High-crime neighborhood and vulnerable client

Driving a mechanically unsafe vehicle

Driving after partaking of alcoholic beverages or drugs

Driving at excessive speeds

Driving without necessary visual aids

Children riding in the front seat in car

Smoking in bed or near oxygen

Overloaded electrical outlets

Grease waste collected on stoves

Use of thin or worn pot holders or mitts

Unrestrained babies riding in car

Nonuse or misuse of seat restraints

Nonuse or misuse of necessary headgear for motorized cyclists or young children carried on adult bicycles

Unsafe road or road-crossing conditions
Play or work near vehicle pathways, e.g., driveways,
lanes, railroad tracks

COMMENTS: Major work is still needed.

Knowledge Deficit (Specify)

† **Definition:** Lack of specific information.
Etiology
    Lack of exposure
    Lack of recall
    Information misinterpretation
    Cognitive limitation
    Lack of interest in learning
    Unfamiliarity with information resources
    † Patient's request for no information
Defining characteristics
    Verbalization of the problem
    Inaccurate follow-through of instruction
    Inadequate performance of test
    Inappropriate or exaggerated behaviors, e.g., hysterical, hostile, agitated, apathetic
    † Statement of misconception
    † Request for information

COMMENTS: Degree of independent nursing therapy:
high.

Mobility, Impaired Physical[1]

Etiology
    Intolerance to activity; decreased strength and endurance

---

[1]Adapted from Jones, E., et al.: Patient classification for long-term care: users' manual, Pub. No. HRA-74-3107, Washington, D.C., Nov. 1974, Department of Health, Education, and Welfare.

Pain and discomfort
Perceptual or cognitive impairment
Neuromuscular impairment
Musculoskeletal impairment
Depression; severe anxiety
Defining characteristics
Inability to purposefully move within the physical environment, including bed mobility, transfer, and ambulation
Reluctance to attempt movement
Limited range of motion
Decreased muscle strength, control, and/or mass
Imposed restrictions of movement, including mechanical; medical protocol
Impaired coordination

COMMENTS: Use of a scale that is applicable when patients are rated from dependence to independence is suggested.
Suggested code for functional level classification
0 Completely independent
1 Requires use of equipment or device
2 Requires help from another person for assistance, supervision, or teaching
3 Requires help from another person and equipment or device
4 Is dependent, does not participate in activity

Noncompliance (Specify)

Definition: Noncompliance is a person's informed decision not to adhere to a therapeutic recommendation.
Etiology
Patient value system
Health beliefs
Cultural influences
Spiritual values
Client and provider relationships

Defining characteristics
   * Behavior indicative of failure to adhere by direct observation or statements by patient or significant others
   Objective tests (physiologic measures, detection of markers)
   Evidence of development of complications
   Evidence of exacerbation of symptoms
   Failure to keep appointments
   Failure to progress
   † Inability to set or attain mutual goals

COMMENTS: Further development and refinement of all areas are needed.

Nutrition, Alteration in: Less Than Body Requirements

Etiology
   Inability to ingest or digest food or absorb nutrients because of biologic, psychologic, or economic factors.
Defining characteristics
   Loss of weight with adequate food intake
   Body weight 20% or more under ideal for height and frame
   Reported inadequate food intake less than RDA[1]
   Weakness of muscles required for swallowing or mastication
   Reported or evidence of lack of food
   Lack of interest in food
   Perceived inability to ingest food
   Aversion to eating
   Reported altered taste sensation
   Satiety immediately after ingesting food
   Abdominal pain with or without pathologic conditions
   Sore, inflamed buccal cavity

---

[1] Recommended daily allowance.

Capillary fragility
Abdominal cramping
Diarrhea and/or steatorrhea
Hyperactive bowel sounds
Pale conjunctiva and mucous membranes
Poor muscle tone
Excessive loss of hair
Lack of information; misinformation
Misconceptions

Nutrition, Alteration in: More Than Body Requirements

Etiology
Excessive intake in relationship to metabolic need
Defining characteristics
Weight 10% over ideal for height and frame
* Weight 20% over ideal for height and frame
* Triceps skin fold greater than 15 mm in men and 25 mm in women
Sedentary activity level
Reported or observed dysfunctional eating patterns
Pairing food with other activities
Concentrating food intake at end of day
Eating in response to external cues such as time of day, social situation
Eating in response to internal cues other than hunger, e.g., anxiety

Nutrition, Alteration in: Potential for More Than Body Requirements

Etiology
Hereditary predisposition
Excessive energy intake during late gestational life, early infancy, and adolescence
Frequent, closely spaced pregnancies
Dysfunctional psychologic conditioning in relationship to food

Membership in lower socioeconomic group

Defining characteristics
* Reported or observed obesity in one or both parents
* Rapid transition across growth percentiles in infants or children

Reported use of solid food as major food source before 5 months of age

Observed use of food as reward or comfort measure

Reported or observed higher baseline weight at beginning of each pregnancy

Dysfunctional eating patterns

Pairing food with other activities

Concentrating food intake at end of day

Eating in response to external cues such as time of day or social situation

Eating in response to internal cues other than hunger such as anxiety

Oral Mucous Membrane, Alteration in

Etiology
Pathologic conditions—oral cavity (radiation to head and/or neck)

Dehydration

Trauma

Chemical, e.g., acidic foods, drugs, noxious agents, alcohol

Mechanical, e.g., ill-fitting dentures, braces, tubes—endotracheal, nasogastric, surgery; oral cavity

NPO instructions for more than 24 hours

Ineffective oral hygiene

Mouth breathing

Malnutrition

Infection

Lack of or decreased salivation

Medication

Defining characteristics
Coated tongue

Xerostomia (dry mouth)
Stomatitis
Oral lesions or ulcers
Lack of or decreased salivation
Leukoplakia
Edema
Hyperemia
Oral plaque
Oral pain or discomfort
Desquamation
Vesicles
Hemorrhagic gingivitis
Carious teeth
Halitosis

COMMENT: New diagnosis

Parenting, Alteration in: Actual or Potential

Definition: Parenting is the ability of a nurturing figure(s) to create an environment that promotes the optimum growth and development of another human being. It is important to state as a preface to this diagnosis that adjustment to parenting in general is a normal maturational process that elicits nursing behaviors of prevention of potential problems and health promotion.

Etiology
Lack of available role model
Ineffective role model
Physical and psychosocial abuse of nurturing figure
Lack of support between or from significant other(s)
Unmet social and emotional maturation needs of parenting figures
Interruption in bonding process, i.e., maternal, paternal, other
Perceived threat to own survival: physical and emotional
Mental and/or physical illness

Presence of stress: financial or legal problems, recent crisis, cultural move

Lack of knowledge

Limited cognitive functioning

Lack of role identity

Lack of appropriate response of child to relationship

Multiple pregnancies

Unrealistic expectation for self, infant, partner

Defining characteristics

Actual and potential

Lack of parental attachment behaviors[1]

Inappropriate visual, tactile, auditory stimulation

Negative identification of characteristics of infant/child

Negative attachment of meanings to characteristics of infant/child

Constant verbalization of disappointment in gender or physical characteristics of infant/child

Verbalization of resentment toward infant/child

Verbalization of role inadequacy

* Inattention to infant/child needs

Verbal disgust at body functions of infant/child

Noncompliance with health appointments for self and/or infant/child

* Inappropriate caretaking behaviors (toilet training, sleep and rest, feeding)

Inappropriate or inconsistent discipline practices

Frequent accidents

Frequent illness

Growth and development lag in the child

* History of child abuse or abandonment by primary caretaker

Verbalizes desire to have child call parent by first name despite traditional cultural tendencies

Child receives care from multiple caretakers without consideration for the needs of the child

Compulsive seeking of role approval from others

Actual
    Abandonment[1]
    Runaway
    Verbalization cannot control child[1]
    Evidence of physical and psychological trauma[1]

COMMENTS: Need to differentiate actual and potential. Further research is needed to identify critical defining characteristics.

Powerlessness

Definition: The perception of the individual that one's own action will not significantly affect an outcome. Powerlessness is the perceived lack of control over a current situation or immediate happening.

Etiology
    Health care environment
    Interpersonal interaction
    Illness-related regimen
    Life-style of helplessness

Defining characteristics
    Severe
        Verbal expressions of having no control or influence over situation
        Verbal expressions of having no control or influence over outcome
        Verbal expressions of having no control over self-care
        Depression over physical deterioration that occurs despite patient compliance with regimens
        Apathy
    Moderate
        Nonparticipation in care or decision making when opportunities are provided

---

[1] Highly critical factor.

Expressions of dissatisfaction and frustration over inability to perform previous tasks and/or activities

Does not monitor progress

Expression of doubt regarding role performance

Reluctance to express true feelings, fearing alienation from care givers

Inability to seek information regarding care

Dependence on others that may result in irritability, resentment, anger, and guilt

Does not defend self-care practices when challenged

Passivity

Low

Passivity

Expressions of uncertainty about fluctuating energy levels

COMMENT: New diagnosis

Rape Trauma Syndrome

Definition: Rape is forced and violent sexual penetration against the victim's will and without the victim's consent. The trauma syndrome that develops from an attack or attempted attack includes an acute phase of disorganization of the victim's life-style and a long-term process of reorganization of life-style. This syndrome includes the following three subcomponents: A, B, and C.

A. RAPE TRAUMA

Defining characteristics

Acute phase

Emotional reactions

Anger

Embarrassment

Fear of physical violence and death

Humiliation

Revenge

Self-blame

Multiple physical symptoms
Gastrointestinal irritability
Genitourinary discomfort
Muscle tension
Sleep pattern disturbance
Long-term phase
Changes in life-style (changes in residence; dealing with repetitive nightmares and phobias; seeking family support; seeking social network support)

B. COMPOUND REACTION

Defining characteristics
All defining characteristics listed under rape trauma
Reactivated symptoms of such previous conditions, i.e., physical illness, psychiatric illness
Reliance on alcohol and/or drugs

C. SILENT REACTION

Defining characteristics
Abrupt changes in relationship with men
Increase in nightmares
Increasing anxiety during interview, i.e., blocking of associations, long periods of silence, minor stuttering, physical distress
Marked changes in sexual behavior
No verbalization of the occurrence of rape
Sudden onset of phobic reactions

Self-Care Deficit: Feeding, Bathing/Hygiene, Dressing/Grooming, Toileting

Etiology
Intolerance to activity; decreased strength and endurance
Pain, discomfort
Perceptual or cognitive impairment
Neuromuscular impairment

Musculoskeletal impairment
Depression; severe anxiety

A. SELF-FEEDING DEFICIT (LEVELS 0 TO 4)[1]
Defining characteristics
Inability to bring food from a receptacle to the mouth

B. SELF-BATHING/HYGIENE (LEVELS 0 TO 4)[1]
Defining characteristics
* Inability to wash body or body parts
Inability to obtain or get to water source
Inability to regulate temperature or flow

C. SELF-DRESSING/GROOMING DEFICIT (LEVELS 0 TO 4)[1]
Defining characteristics
* Impaired ability to put on or take off necessary items of clothing
Impaired ability to obtain or replace articles of clothing
Impaired ability to fasten clothing
Inability to maintain appearance at a satisfactory level

D. SELF-TOILETING DEFICIT (LEVELS 0 TO 4)[1]
Etiology (broad categories)
Impaired transfer ability
Impaired mobility status
Intolerance to activity; decreased strength and endurance
Pain, discomfort
Perceptual or cognitive impairment
Neuromuscular impairment
Musculoskeletal impairment
Depression, severe anxiety
Defining characteristics
* Unable to get to toilet or commode
* Unable to sit on or rise from toilet or commode

---

[1] For definition of code see Mobility, impaired physical.

* Unable to manipulate clothing for toileting
* Unable to carry out proper toilet hygiene
Unable to flush toilet or empty commode

Self-concept, Disturbance in: Body Image, Self-esteem, Role Performance, Personal Identity

Definition: A disturbance in self-concept is a disruption in the way one perceives one's body image, self-esteem, role performance, and/or personal identity. These four subcomponents, in turn, have their own etiologies and defining characteristics (Figure 1).

A. BODY IMAGE, DISTURBANCE IN

Etiology

    Biophysical
    Cognitive perceptual
    Psychosocial
    Cultural or spiritual

Defining characteristics

Either the following A or B must be present to justify the diagnosis of body image, alteration in:

    *A. Verbal response to actual or perceived change in structure and/or function
    *B. Nonverbal response to actual or perceived change in structure and/or function

The following clinical manifestations may be used to validate the presence of A or B:

    Objective
        Missing body part
        Actual change in structure and/or function
        Not looking at body part
        Not touching body part
        Hiding or overexposing body part (intentional or unintentional)
        Trauma to nonfunctioning part
        Change in social involvement

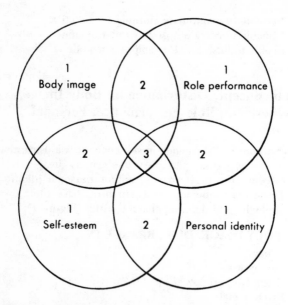

Figure 1. Defining characteristics of a disturbance in self-concepts are (1) critical characteristic or cluster of characteristics specific to the subcategory, (2) characteristic or cluster of characteristics shared by subcategories but not common to all subcategories, and (3) characteristic or cluster of characteristics common to all subcategories. (From Kim, M.J., and Moritz, D.A., editors: Classification of nursing diagnoses: proceedings of the Third and Fourth National Conferences, New York, 1982, McGraw-Hill Book Co., p. 308.)

Change in ability to estimate spatial relationship of
    body to environment
Subjective
Verbalization of
    Change in life-style
    Fear of rejection or of reaction by others
    Focus on past strength, function, or appearance

Negative feelings about body
Feelings of helplessness, hopelessness, or powerlessness
Preoccupation with change or loss
Emphasis on remaining strengths, heightened achievement
Extension of body boundary to incorporate environmental objects
Personalization of part or loss by name
Depersonalization of part or loss by impersonal pronouns
Refusal to verify actual change

Degree of independent nursing therapy (this may be related to etiology):
Biophysical: low degree of nursing independence
Psychosocial: medium to high degree of nursing independence
Cognitive perceptual: high degree of nursing independence
Cultural spiritual: medium to high degree of nursing independence
It may be possible to identify high-risk populations, such as those with following conditions:
Missing parts
Dependence on machine
Significance of body part or functioning with regard to age, sex, developmental level, or basic human needs
Physical change caused by biochemical agents (drugs)
Physical trauma or mutilation
Pregnancy and/or maturational changes

B. SELF-ESTEEM, DISTURBANCE IN

Etiology
To be developed
Defining characteristics
Inability to accept positive reinforcement
Lack of follow-through

Nonparticipation in therapy
Not taking responsibility for self-care (self-neglect)
Self-destructive behavior
Lack of eye contact

C. ROLE PERFORMANCE, DISTURBANCE IN

Etiology
  To be developed
Defining characteristics
  Change in self-perception of role
  Denial of role
  Change in others' perception of role
  Conflict in roles
  Change in physical capacity to resume role
  Lack of knowledge of role
  Change in usual patterns or responsibility

D. PERSONAL IDENTITY, DISTURBANCE IN

Definition: Inability to distinguish between self and non-self.
Etiology
  To be developed
Defining characteristics
  To be developed

COMMENTS: Further development in the following areas is recommended:
  1. Define and develop each of the four subsets of self-esteem, body image, role performance, and personal identity.
  2. Develop etiologies and characteristics for the four subset areas.
  3. Identify most commonly shared characteristics of the four subset areas.
  4. Use previously documented work (as included in this section) as a basis for further development.
  5. Consider including such components as "group relations, noneffective" and "sexuality."

Sensory-Perceptual Alteration: Visual, Auditory, Kinesthetic, Gustatory, Tactile, Olfactory

Etiology

†The etiological statement should be expanded to include the following:

Environmental factors

   Therapeutically restricted environments (isolation, intensive care, bedrest, traction, confining illnesses, incubator)

   Socially restricted environment (institutionalization, home-bound, aging, chronic illness, dying, infant deprivation); stigmatized (mentally ill, mentally retarded, mentally handicapped); bereaved

Altered sensory reception, transmission, and/or integration

   Neurologic disease, trauma, or deficit

   Altered status of sense organs

   Inability to communicate, understand, speak, or respond

   Sleep deprivation

   Pain

Chemical alteration

   Endogenous (eletrolyte imbalance, elevated BUN, elevated ammonia, hypoxia)

   Exogenous (central nervous system stimulants or depressants, mind-altering drugs)

Psychologic stress (narrowed perceptual fields caused by anxiety)

Defining characteristics

Disoriented in time, in place, or with persons

Altered abstraction

Altered conceptualization

Change in problem-solving abilities

Reported or measured change in sensory acuity

Change in behavior pattern

Anxiety

Apathy
Change in usual response to stimuli
Indication of body-image alteration
Restlessness
Irritability
Altered communication patterns
†Disorientation
†Lack of concentration
†Daydreaming
†Hallucinations
†Noncompliance
†Fear
†Depression
†Rapid mood swings
†Anger
†Exaggerated emotional responses
†Poor concentration
†Disordered thought sequencing
†Bizarre thinking
†Visual and auditory distortions
†Motor incoordination
Other possible defining characteristics
Complaints of fatigue
Alteration in posture
Change in muscular tension
Inappropriate responses
Hallucinations

Sexual Dysfunction

Etiology
Biopsychosocial alteration of sexuality
Ineffectual or absent role models
Physical abuse
Psychosocial abuse, e.g., harmful relationships
Vulnerability
Misinformation or lack of knowledge
Values conflict
Lack of privacy

Lack of significant other
Altered body structure or function: pregnancy, recent childbirth, drugs, surgery, anomalies, disease process, trauma, radiation

Defining characteristics
Verbalization of problem
Alterations in achieving perceived sex role
Actual or perceived limitation imposed by disease and/or therapy
Conflicts involving values
Alterations in achieving sexual satisfaction
Inability to achieve desired satisfaction
Seeking of confirmation of desirability
Alteration in relationship with significant other
Change of interest in self and others

Skin Integrity, Impairment of: Actual

Etiology
External (environmental)
Hyperthermia or hypothermia
Chemical substance
Mechanical factors
Shearing forces
Pressure
Restraint
Radiation
Physical immobilization
Humidity
Internal (somatic)
Medication
Altered nutritional state: obesity, emaciation
Altered metabolic state
Altered circulation
Altered sensation
Altered pigmentation
Skeletal prominence
Developmental factors
Immunologic deficit

Alterations in turgor (change in elasticity)
†Excretions/secretions
†Psychogenic
†Edema
Defining characteristics
  Disruption of skin surface
  Destruction of skin layers
  Invasion of body structures

Skin Integrity, Impairment of: Potential

Etiology
  Not applicable
Defining characteristics[1]
  External (environmental)
    Hypothermia or hyperthermia
    Chemical substance
    Mechanical factors
      Shearing forces
      Pressure
      Restraint
    Radiation
    Physical immobilization
    Excretions and secretions
    Humidity
  Internal (somatic)
    Medication
    Alterations in nutritional state (obesity, emaciation)
    Altered metabolic state
    Altered circulation
    Altered sensation
    Altered pigmentation
    Skeletal prominence
    Developmental factors
    Alterations in skin turgor (change in elasticity)

---

[1] Presence of one or more risk factors (something that increases the possibility of a condition occurring).

Psychogenic
Immunologic

COMMENTS: This diagnosis remains the same as that of 1978, but the group recommended further development.

Sleep Pattern Disturbance

Definition: Disruption of sleep time which causes patient discomfort or interferes with the patient's desired life-style.

Etiology
Sensory alterations
Internal factors
Illness
Psychologic stress
External factors
Environmental changes
Social cues

Defining characteristics
*Verbal complaints of difficulty in falling asleep
*Awakening earlier or later than desired
*Interrupted sleep
*Verbal complaints of not feeling well rested
Changes in behavior and performance
Increasing irritability
Restlessness
Disorientation
Lethargy
Listlessness
Physical signs
Mild, fleeting nystagmus
Slight hand tremor
Ptosis of eyelid
Expressionless face
Thick speech with mispronunciation and incorrect words

Dark circles under eyes
Frequent yawning
Changes in posture
†Not feeling well rested

Social Isolation

Definition: Condition of aloneness experienced by the individual and perceived as imposed by others and as a negative or threatened state.

Etiology

Factors contributing to the absence of satisfying personal relationships, such as the following:

Delay in accomplishing developmental tasks
Immature interests
Alterations in physical appearance
Alterations in mental status
Unaccepted social behavior
Unaccepted social values
Altered state of wellness
Inadequate personal resources
Inability to engage in satisfying personal relationships

Defining characteristics

Objective

Absence of supportive significant other(s)—family, friends, group
Sad, dull affect
Inappropriate or immature interests & activities for developmental age or stage
Uncommunicative, withdrawn; no eye contact
Preoccupation with own thoughts; repetitive, meaningless actions
Projects hostility in voice, behavior
Seeks to be alone or exists in subculture
Evidence of physical and/or mental handicap or altered state of wellness
Shows behavior unaccepted by dominant cultural group

Subjective

Expresses feeling of aloneness imposed by others

Expresses feelings of rejection

Experiences feelings of difference from others

Expresses values acceptable to subculture, but unable to accept values of dominant culture

Inadequacy in or absence of significant purpose in life

Inability to meet expectations of others

Insecurity in public

Expresses interests inappropriate to developmental age or stage

COMMENT: New diagnosis

Spiritual Distress (Distress of the Human Spirit)

Definition: Distress of the human spirit is a disruption in the life principle that pervades a person's entire being and that integrates and transcends one's biologic and psychosocial nature.

Etiology

Separation from religious and cultural ties

Challenged belief and value system, e.g., result of moral or ethical implications of therapy or result of intense suffering

Defining characteristics

*Expresses concern with meaning of life and death and/or belief systems

Anger toward God (as defined by the person)

Questions meaning of suffering

Verbalizes inner conflict about beliefs

Verbalizes concern about relationship with deity

Questions meaning for own existence

Unable to choose or chooses not to participate in usual religious practices

Seeks spiritual assistance

Questions moral and ethical implications of therapeutic regimen

Displacement of anger toward religious representatives

Description of nightmares or sleep disturbances

Alteration in behavior or mood evidenced by anger, crying, withdrawal, preoccupation, anxiety, hostility, apathy, etc.

†Regards illness as punishment

†Does not experience that God is forgiving

†Unable to accept self

†Engages in self-blame

†Denies responsibilities for problems

†Description of somatic complaints

COMMENTS: The following more specific diagnostic labels (including corresponding etiologies) along with defining characteristics are more fully discussed in Chapter 6 of the Proceedings[1]: spiritual distress related to forgiveness, spiritual distress related to love, spiritual distress related to hope, spiritual distress related to trust, and spiritual distress related to meaning and purpose in life.

Thought Processes, Alteration in

Etiology
†Physiologic changes
†Psychologic conflicts
†Loss of memory
†Impaired judgment
†Sleep deprivation

Defining characteristics
Inaccurate interpretation of environment

---

[1]Kim, M. J., McLane, A. M., and McFarland, G. K., editors: Classification of nursing diagnosis: proceedings of The Fifth National Conference, St. Louis, 1984, The C. V. Mosby Co.

Cognitive dissonance
Distractibility
Memory deficit or problems
Egocentricity
Hyper/hypovigilance
†Decreased ability to grasp ideas
†Impaired ability to make decisions
†Impaired ability to problem solve
†Impaired ability to reason
†Impaired ability to abstract or conceptualize
†Impaired ability to calculate
†Altered attention span—distractibility
†Commands; obsessions
†Inability to follow
†Disorientation to time, place, person, circumstances, and events
†Changes in remote, recent, immediate memory
†Delusions
†Ideas of reference
†Hallucinations
†Confabulation
†Inappropriate social behavior
†Altered sleep patterns
†Inappropriate affect
Other possible defining characteristics
Inappropriate/nonreality-based thinking

Tissue Perfusion, Alteration in: Cerebral, Cardiopulmonary, Renal, Gastrointestinal, Peripheral

Etiology
Interruption of flow, arterial
Interruption of flow, venous
Exchange problems
Hypervolemia
Hypovolemia

Defining characteristics	Chances of defining characteristic being present in given diagnosis	Chances of defining characteristic not being explained by any other diagnosis
Skin temperature cold extremities	High	Low
Skin color		
Dependent, blue or purple	Moderate	Low
*Pale on elevation, and color does not return on lowering leg	High	High
*Diminished arterial pulsations	High	High
Skin quality: shining	High	Low
Lack of lanugo	High	Moderate
Round scars covered with atrophied skin		
Gangrene	Low	High
Slow-growing, dry, thick brittle nails	High	Moderate
Claudication	Moderate	High
Blood pressure changes in extremities		
Bruits	Moderate	Moderate
Slow healing of lesions	High	Low

COMMENTS: Further work and development are required for the five subcomponents of this diagnosis, specifically cerebral, renal, and gastrointestinal.

Urinary Elimination, Alteration in Patterns
Etiology
Sensory motor impairment

†Neuromuscular impairment
†Mechanical trauma
Defining characteristics
  Dysuria
  Frequency
  Hesitancy
  Incontinence
  Nocturia
  Retention
  Urgency

COMMENTS: Previous etiologies—anatonomic obstruction and urinary tract infection—were eliminated.

Violence, Potential for: Self-Directed or Directed at Others

Etiology
  Antisocial character
  Battered women
  Catatonic excitement
  Child abuse
  Manic excitement
  Organic brain syndrome
  Panic states
  Rage reactions
  Suicidal behavior
  Temporal lobe epilepsy
  Toxic reactions to medication
Defining characteristics
  Body language: clenched fists, facial expressions, rigid posture, tautness indicating intense effort to control
  Hostile threatening verbalizations; boasting of prior abuse to others
  Increased motor activity, pacing, excitement, irritability, agitation
  Overt and aggressive acts; goal-directed destruction of objects in environment

Possession of destructive means; gun, knife, weapon

Rage

Self-destructive behavior and/or active, aggressive suicidal acts

Substance abuse or withdrawal

Suspicion of others, paranoid ideation, delusions, hallucinations

Other defining characteristics

Increasing anxiety level

Fear of self or others

Inability to verbalize feelings

Repetition of verbalizations: continues complaints, requests, and demands

Anger

Provocative behavior: argumentative, dissatisfied, overreactive, hypersensitive

Vulnerable self-esteem

Depression (specifically active, aggressive, suicidal acts)

List of Nursing Diagnoses Accepted at the Third National Conference

Adjustment to illness, impairment of significant others

Anxiety, mild

Anxiety, moderate

Anxiety, severe

Anxiety, panic

Body fluids, excess

Bowel elimination, alteration in: constipation

Bowel elimination, alteration in: diarrhea

Bowel elimination, alteration in: impaction

Bowel elimination, alteration in: incontinence

Cardiac output, alteration in: decreased

Circulation, interruption of

Comfort, alteration in: pain

Communication, impaired verbal

Consciousness, altered levels of
Coping patterns, family, ineffective
Coping patterns, individual, maladaptive
Fluid volume deficit, actual (1,2)
Fluid volume deficit, potential
Functional performance, variations in
Functional performance, variations in: home mainte-
nance management impaired
Grieving
Injury, potential for
Injury: susceptibility to hazard
Knowledge, lack of (specify as to area)
Mobility, impairment of
Noncompliance
Nutrition, alterations in: less than body requirements
Nutrition, alterations in: more than body requirements
Nutrition, alterations in: changes related to body re-
quirements
Parenting, alterations in: actual or potential
Respiratory dysfunction
Self-care activities, alteration in: ability to perform hy-
giene
Self-concept, alteration in: body image, self-esteem, role
performance, personal identity
Sensory-perceptual alterations
Sexuality, alteration in patterns of
Skin integrity, impairment of: actual
Skin integrity, impairment of: potential
Sleep/rest activity, dysrhythm of
Spirituality: spiritual concerns
Spirituality: spiritual distress
Spirituality: spiritual despair
Thought processes impaired
Tissue perfusion, abnormal, chronic
Urinary elimination, impairment of: alteration in pat-
terns
Urinary elimination, impairment of: incontinence
Urinary elimination, impairment of: retention

Prototype care plans using nursing diagnoses*

---

*Defining characteristics of the diagnoses presented here are the same as those listed in Section II.

NURSING CARE OF PATIENTS WITH CARDIOVASCULAR PROBLEMS

Cardiac output, alteration in: decreased

Margaret J. Stafford, R.N., M.S.N., F.A.A.N., and Meg Gulanick, R.N., M.S.

Etiology	Goals	Nursing intervention	Outcome criteria
Alteration in preload, afterload, heart rate, contractility, or conduction disturbance	Optimal hemodynamic function	Assess physical status as appropriate, monitor and document changes, report significant alterations (vital signs, heart and lung sounds; jugular vein distention; skin; fluid balance) Monitor ECG for rate, rhythm, and ectopy. If arrhythmia occurs, determine patient response, document, report to physician as appropriate, and treat according to protocol.	Following measurements will return toward patient's optimal level: Hemodynamic measures (e.g., BP PAP, PCWP, CVP, MAP) Electrical conduction of the heart

Administer medications and fluids as ordered, noting effectiveness and side effects.	Physical activity level
Adjust patient's activity to reduce O_2 demands. Provide rest periods.	Urinary output
Monitor therapeutic aids within prescribed protocol (pacemaker, intraaortic balloon, etc.)	Mental status
Maintain adequate perfusion (oxygen, positioning, etc.)	
Implement emergency measures based on nursing judgment on protocol.	

NURSING CARE OF PATIENTS WITH CARDIOVASCULAR PROBLEMS

Alteration in comfort, chest pain

By Margaret J. Stafford, R.N., M.S.N., F.A.A.N., and Meg Gulanick, R.N., M.S.

Etiology	Goals	Nursing intervention	Outcome criteria
Altered myocardial oxygen supply	Relief or minimization of pain, improved comfort	Assess presence or absence of pain. If present, assess pain characteristics (duration, quality, location, etc.)	Relief of pain or minimization of pain as evidenced by verbalization and appearance of relief of pain
		Anticipate need for analgesics and/or additional methods of pain relief (e.g., O_2 administration, possible stress relief)	
		Respond immediately to pain complaints; report to physician as appropriate	
		Record 12-lead ECG during chest pain as appropriate; monitor changes in ST segment, T wave, and pattern of chest pain; assess and report to physician when pain is not relieved by nitroglycerin administration	
		Provide rest periods to decrease O_2 demands	

NURSING CARE OF SCHOOL CHILDREN IN THE COMUNITY
Health maintenance, alteration (community)* —regarding dental care

Dorothea F. Jakob, R.N., M.S.N.

Intermediate nursing goal: the next school dental survey will show a 50% decrease in the approximately 250 children who were last identified as having untreated caries, neglected hygiene, or periodontal disease.

Etiology	Goals	Nursing intervention	Outcome criteria
Student and family knowledge deficits regarding The importance of primary teeth vis-a-vis secondary teeth The elements of basic dental prevention and reasonable self-care maintenance behaviors	Students and parents will become the focus of an educational effort regarding healthy teeth, dental care, prevention and resources	Offer brief teaching and support to children in this group with untreated caries Send home dental information along with each request for parental permission for DPH dental care	Each child in the identified group will have begun dental treatment for caries in this school year Older children with excellent dental knowledge will be identified and become school resources

*Community in focus: the 700 children of an inner-city elementary school and their families.

Continued.

69

NURSING CARE OF SCHOOL CHILDREN IN THE COMMUNITY—cont'd
Health maintenance, alteration (community)—regarding dental care

Etiology	Goals	Nursing intervention	Outcome criteria
The existence of tax-supported, health department (DPH) dental and hygienist services and how to use them, secondary to		Facilitate multidisciplinary teaching efforts	The DPH hygienist will maximize this school's teaching program
Misconceptions, lack of exposure and information nonuse		Request complimentary tooth brushes and paste from various companies	During dental week each child in the group will be given a toothbrush and paste
Language and educational barriers on the part of parents, written dental notices sent home, and follow-up by staff	The parents or guardians will be able to understand written materials regarding care that are sent home	Request translations of dental information materials	Any information sent home will be direct and straightforward be translated into the language read by the parents/guardians

Unavailable adults to accompany children to dental resources, secondary to	Children of parents who have given permission for DPH dental care will be adequately accompanied to the clinics and given emotional support	Request parental permission for DPH care for children in this group with caries	The school staff will coordinate adult accompaniment for children under 11 years
Economic and energy priorities of struggling, blue collar, immigrant families regarding work absenteeism or private dental care		Role model the importance of adult accompaniment and support for children under 11 years having DPH dental care	Public health nurse will coordinate the buddy system with teacher assistance
		Request the principal to help problem solve the need for further adult accompaniment	
		Institute a buddy system for responsible 13-year-olds to accompany 11-13 year old children	
Knowledge deficit and uncoordinated efforts by the many school and DPH personnel concerning the scope and severity of the problem	Knowledge concerning the scope and etiology of the problem and the difficulties in the systems will become the basis for multidisciplinary collaboration of efforts	Share all information with the principal	Teachers will be urged to include a dental teaching unit in each classes' curriculum
		Explore various alternatives for enhancing the DPH dental resources for the school	The DPH dental treatment hours will be expanded to meet the needs of this school

Continued.

NURSING CARE OF SCHOOL CHILDREN IN THE COMMUNITY—cont'd

Health maintenance, alteration (community)—regarding dental care

Etiology	Goals	Nursing intervention	Outcome criteria
		Facilitate collaboration of DPH and school resources and personnel	The school teaching program will include multidisciplinary activities
			Communications among the dental clinics, the hygienist, and the school will increase
Avoidance tactics by children fearful of uncomfortable dental treatment	Fearful children will receive dental care with minimal trauma	Offer brief teaching and support to children for whom dental care is a priority	Fear and discomfort will be acknowledged frankly and will not sabotage the children's corrective care
		Offer more intensive support and teaching to clearly fearful children	
		Arrange the most feasible, supportive accompaniment for children using DPH dental services	

NURSING CARE OF CLIENTS IN THE COMMUNITY
Home maintenance management, impaired

Dorothea F. Jakob, R.N., M.S.N.

Overall nursing goal: Enable the client to continue living at home as long as it is safe and desired

Etiology	Goals	Nursing intervention	Outcome criteria
Unorganized (or absent) support system	Support system will contribute in maximum, realistic ways to help maintain the client at home	Assess system capacities Assist with system planning and organizing Offer emotional and practical assistance to the system	Support system members will Offer specific, regular contributions to help maintain the client Outreach for assistance when necessary
Insufficient use of community resources secondary to Knowledge deficit of them	The client will choose to make use of appropriate community resources	Facilitate recognition of the need for additional resources in the home Share information regarding appropriate resources Facilitate problem-solving process	Community resources for home or meal assistance and social stimulation, etc., will Be known by the client

Originally submitted by Dorothea Fox Jakob (with etiology and defining characteristics) to the Third National Conference; see Kim, M.J., and Moritz, D.A.: Classification of nursing diagnoses: proceedings of the Third and Fourth National Conferences, New York, 1982, McGraw-Hill Book Co., p. 293. *Continued.*

NURSING CARE OF CLIENTS IN THE COMMUNITY—cont'd

Home maintenance management, impaired

Overall nursing goal: Enable the client to continue living at home as long as it is safe and desired

Etiology	Goals	Nursing intervention	Outcome criteria
Decreased outreach to them		Facilitate direct outreach or referral to chosen resources on a trial basis	Be appropriately used by the client
Decreased cognitive functioning			
Financial insufficiencies			
Decreasing physical energy resources secondary to	The client will attain a maximum, realistic level of compensation to pathologic conditions present	Facilitate interdisciplinary assessment of activity tolerance, range of motion, and realistic activity goals	Physical activity will Be augmented by specified range of motion or other exercise
Activity intolerances of normal aging and pathology present	The client will enhance his or her level of safe activity tolerance	Encourage and demonstrate realistic exercises; refer to an existing rehabilitation resource if appropriate	Be modulated by adequate rest, sleep, and nutritional pattern
Insufficient physical exercise		Facilitate recognition of the need and planning for adequate activity/task/rest pattern	
Insufficient nutritional intake			

Ineffective energy planning and establishing of task priorities	The client will increase nutritional intake to an acceptable level		Be done on a planned basis according to priorities
	The client's activity-rest pattern will enable maximum activities of daily living		
Dysfunctional grieving	The client will show progress with grief work and resolution of depression	Validate the identified losses and personal impact of grief	The client will: Share feeling of loss with at least one other person
		Encourage ventilation	Appreciate the importance of his or her grief work
		Encourage sharing with a sensitized significant other or professional resource; offer support to the significant other	Recognize progress in his or her grief
		Work through depressive feelings	Demonstrate progress in resolving depression

NURSING CARE OF PATIENTS WITH DEVELOPMENTAL DISABILITIES

Bowel elimination, alteration in: constipation

Jacqueline Miller, R.N., M.S., and Kathlyn Steele, R.N., M.S.

Etiology	Goals	Nursing intervention*	Outcome criteria
Blended or liquid diet consistency	Will require no more than four suppositories per month within 3 months	For individuals who take food and fluids by mouth	Fluid intake equals established amounts
Gavage feedings		1. Prunes (4 oz) daily at breakfast	Stools softer in consistency
Spasticity	Will eliminate soft-formed stool every 3 days without aid of laxatives	2. Bran (4 tsp) in breakfast cereal daily	Decreased dependency on laxatives, enemas, or suppositories compared to baseline
Immobility		3. 1 oz bread crumbs for fiber (add to blended food to thicken)	
Inadequate fluid intake		4. Bulk laxatives, enemas, suppositories per physician's order	
Poor muscle tonicity (atonic bowel)	Will require no more than one enema per month in 6 months	5. Minimum amount of fluid intake daily as ordered	Spontaneous eliminations on a more regular basis
Skeletal deformities		6. Fresh fruits, raw vegetables in diet daily	
Side effect of anticonvulsants		7. Gel juices, milk gel, increased fluid content	
Dependence on laxatives, suppositories, or enemas			

76

Lack of exercise	8. Position change every hour during waking hours and every 2 hours at night
	9. Placed on stool, commode, or bedpan after breakfast for 15–20 minutes daily
	For individuals who take food and fluids by gavage
	1. Prune juice (4 oz) at 10 AM daily
	2. Bulk laxatives, enemas, suppositories per physician's order
	3. Minimum amount of fluid intake daily as ordered
	4. Position change every hour during waking hours and every 2 hours at night
	5. Placed on stool, commode, or bedpan after breakfast for 15–20 minutes daily

*Physician's order or protocol may be necessary for the implementation of some nursing interventions.

NURSING CARE OF PATIENTS WITH DEVELOPMENTAL DISABILITIES
Nutrition, alteration in: less than body requirements

Jacqueline Miller, R.N., M.S.

Etiology	Goals	Nursing intervention*	Outcome criteria
Vomiting	Will retain meals at least 30 minutes after eating	For the individual who is able to take foods orally	Weight gained or maintained as determined
Rumination		1. Referral to dietician for evaluation of nutritional status and assessment	
Malabsorption syndrome	Will gain 2 pounds per month to a maximum of 10–12 pounds in 6 months		Meals retained more than 30 minutes
Poor sucking and swallowing		2. Weigh weekly on Tuesday at 6:30 AM in pajamas for 3 months	Episodes of vomiting and rumination reduced in frequency and amount
Malocclusion	Will maintain appropriate weight for height in 3 months (identify weight range specific for individual)	3. Elevate head of bed and maintain upright at least 30 minutes after eating	Increased interest in the eating process
Hyperactive and hypoactive gag reflexes		4. Position in adaptive chair for at least 30 minutes after eating	Increased variety of foods tolerated and consumed
High arched palate		5. Feed in a calm and unhurried manner	
Tongue thrust			
Failure to thrive		6. Increase caloric intake to amount of calories per body weight as ordered	Increased energy level
Gastritis			
Esophageal strictures			

Hiatal hernia
Decreased appetite
Lethargy from anti-
convulsants
Spasticity

Increased distractible
behavior at mealtimes
Food allergies
Lactose intolerance

7. Offer six small feedings daily at
   7, 1, 4, 7, and 10 o'clock
8. Document all episodes of food
   refusal, portions eaten, food loss
   or vomiting, spitting out, rumi-
   nation
9. High-caloric breakfast of cream
   and honey
10. Bedtime snack of high-caloric
    pudding
11. Feeding facilitation techniques
    as needed
12. Offer pacifier to increase suck-
    ing ability
13. Prepare for mealtime—speak in
    a soft tone and explain events
    while feeding
14. Yogurt, gel juices, and milk gels
    added to diet

*Physician's order or protocol may be necessary for the implementation of some nursing interventions.

Continued.

NURSING CARE OF PATIENTS WITH DEVELOPMENTAL DISABILITIES—cont'd
Nutrition, alteration in: less than body requirements

Etiology	Goals	Nursing intervention*	Outcome criteria
		15. Glucose polymer (30 calories/tablespoon) added to diet to increase calories	
		For the individual who receives gavage method of feeding	
		1. Document all episodes of fluid feeding intolerance, vomiting, and rumination	
		2. Feed by gavage (as ordered) for 5 feedings at slow drip with head of bed elevated 30 degrees	
		3. Offer small amounts of blended food at each meal by mouth	
		4. Oral hygiene measures include brushing and mouth washes between feedings	

5. Flavored lip lubrication following oral hygiene

6. Feeding facilitation techniques for oral stimulation at 10, 1, and 6 o'clock

7. Refer to dietician for evaluation of nutritional status and assessment

8. Weigh weekly on Tuesday at 6:30 AM in pajamas for 3 months

9. Elevate head of bed and maintain upright at least 30 minutes after eating

10. Position in adaptive chair for at least 30 minutes after eating

11. Increase caloric intake to amount of calories per body weight as ordered

12. Prepare for mealtime—speak in a soft tone and explain events while feeding

NURSING CARE OF PATIENTS WITH DIABETES
Knowledge deficit (insulin administration)
Pamela Gotch, R.N., M.S.N.

Etiology	Goals	Nursing intervention	Outcome criteria
Lack of prior exposure to the procedure	To increase knowledge and skill regarding insulin administration	Assess eyesight, manual dexterity, memory, and simple mathematical abilities in relation to the skills required for insulin self-administration	Patient and/or significant other is able to
Misinterpretation of information received in the past		Instruct patient and/or significant other on the importance of following prescribed insulin regimen at home	Verbalize the name, dosage, concentration, and action times of the prescribed insulin
Inability to recall information received in the past		Explain name, dosage, concentration, and action times of prescribed insulin and the relationship of timing to the patient's meal schedule	Verbalize the schedule for insulin and its relation to meals.
Past inability to invest self in learning the procedure		Initiate insulin instructions by preparing all insulin at patient's bedside	Verbalize the importance of using syringes that correspond to the concentration of the insulin prescribed (U-40 or U-100)

Provide patient and/or significant other with syringes, alcohol wipes, and sterile water as practice materials; use the same equipment as will be used at home	Verbalize the care, expiration date, storage, disposal, and purchasing of insulin and syringes (including sterilization of glass syringe if used)
Use written instruction sheets to supplement verbal instruction	Verbalize travel tips for insulin therapy
Consider having the patient perform only part of the procedure at one given time (drawing up only or injecting only); advance patient to drawing up and giving all of own insulin with supervision	Demonstrate the ability to accurately withdraw and administer prescribed dose(s) of insulin
Confer with physicians regarding their preference for injection sites	
Discuss importance of site rotation; set up site rotation chart that patient can use at home	

Continued.

NURSING CARE OF PATIENTS WITH DIABETES—cont'd
Knowledge deficit (insulin administration)

Etiology	Goals	Nursing intervention	Outcome criteria
		Plan for a *minimum* of three self-administrations before discharge; plan for one injection in the abdomen, if not contraindicated	Demonstrate the ability to accurately identify and rotate injection sites
		Instruct patient to record injection sites on site rotation chart	Demonstrate ability to maintain site rotation chart
		Instruct patient and/or significant other on the importance of purchasing the same concentration of insulin and corresponding syringes	Verbalize that insulin dose(s) must be taken everyday
		Explain proper care, expiration date, storage, purchasing, and disposal of insulin and syringes; if glass syringes are used, instruct on sterilization procedure	

If appropriate to patient's current life-style, review travel tips pertinent to insulin therapy

If patient is not able to draw up and/or inject own insulin, provide opportunities for significant others to demonstrate skill

Instruct significant other on prefilling syringes if appropriate

Provide patient with supplies at time of discharge

Assess patient's confidence in own ability to self-administer insulin at home; arrange for community health referral if necessary to build a sense of competence

NURSING CARE OF PATIENTS WITH DIABETES
Skin integrity, impairment of: potential
Pamela Gotch, R.N., M.S.N.

Etiology	Goals	Nursing intervention	Outcome criteria
Decreased circulation	Prevent skin breakdown	Assess condition of patient's skin, especially feet	Skin integrity maintained
Diminished sensation		Identify the risk factors that are present	Toenails are properly trimmed prior to discharge
Increased susceptibility to infection		Institute appropriate skin and foot care routine while patient is hospitalized	Patient and/or significant other is able to
Knowledge and/or skill deficit regarding preventive measures		If toenails are thickened and/or patient is unable to manage own nail care, confer with physician regarding use of physician or podiatrist for nail care	Verbalize knowledge of the effects of diabetes on circulation, healing, and sensation
Noncompliance to recommended foot care practices		If toenails require trimming, attempt to complete this health need during the time the patient is hospitalized	Demonstrate daily skin and foot care routines
Fluid volume deficit (actual)—altered skin turgor			

Explain to patient and/or significant other special skin and foot care in relation to effects of diabetes on circulation, sensation, and healing	Verbalize knowledge of the measures necessary to protect the integrity of the extremities
Demonstrate proper foot care, including	Verbalize knowledge of the signs and symptoms that warrant notification of physician
1. Daily bathing and drying thoroughly with soft towel (especially between toes)	
2. Foot inspection, including soles of feet and areas between toes	Verbalize knowledge of the appropriate care required for minor injuries and/or other changes
3. Checking temperature of bath water with wrist or elbow rather than with feet	
Have patient reenact the demonstration	
Instruct patient in the proper care of minor injuries, which include	
1. Keeping area clean and dry	
2. Elevating foot as much as possible	
3. Avoiding any further irritation such as pressure or application of caustic antiseptics	

Continued.

NURSING CARE OF PATIENTS WITH DIABETES—cont'd
Skin integrity, impairment of: potential

Etiology	Goals	Nursing intervention	Outcome criteria
		Instruct patient in the signs and symptoms of a developing problem, which include 1. Injury that does not heal 2. Change in color, temperature, or sensation of an extremity 3. Indicators of an infection (redness, swelling, tenderness) Instruct patient to seek prompt medical attention Instruct patient in preventive measures, which include 1. Adequate protection from well-fitting footwear 2. Avoidance of exposure to extremes in temperature 3. Protection from unnecessary chemical or mechanical injury 4. Avoidance of smoking Provide written materials to supplement verbal instructions If patient is unable to manage own foot care, delegate foot care to a responsible significant other and explain as above	

NURSING CARE OF MATERNITY CLIENTS
Knowledge deficit (breast feeding)
Donna Lawrence, R.N., M.S.

Etiology	Goals	Nursing intervention	Outcome criteria
Lack of skill, experience, and knowledge	Increase knowledge base regarding breast-feeding	Encourage verbalization about decision to breast-feed	At the time of hospital discharge mother will
First-time attempt at breast-feeding		Provide environment conducive to breast-feeding	Relate nutritional requisites for lactating mother
Mother unsure whether breast-feeding is her method of choice		Ascertain mother's knowledge level and prenatal preparation for breast-feeding	Demonstrate good food choices through menu review
		Meet mother's comfort needs	
		Discuss scheduling of feedings—adjust hospital routine to needs of infant (allow demand feeding scheduling)	Demonstrate appropriate breast self-care
		Increase time at breast gradually to toughen nipples	

Continued.

NURSING CARE OF MATERNITY CLIENTS—cont'd
Knowledge deficit (breast feeding)

Etiology	Goals	Nursing intervention	Outcome criteria
		Discuss and allow mother to assume breast self-care: Nipple care Use of ointment Air drying Use of heat Review nutritional and fluid requirements for lactating mothers Provide written guides for food choices Teach guidelines for successful breast-feeding: Rooting Positions (cradle, lying, football) Nipple placement Breaking suction Supply and demand Let-down phenomena Emptying all breast ducts Treatment of nipple soreness	Demonstrate skill with breast feeding, use of alternate positions Display increased comfort in role as determined by body language Be able to manually and mechanically express breast milk Relate signs and symptoms of infant satiety Discuss need for increased rest with realistic plans for same at home

Demonstrate hand expression of milk from breast—provide mother with opportunity to perform procedure	Recognize normal stools of infant who is breast-fed
Discuss mechanical breast pumps and their use	Have determined that breast-feeding is her method of choice for feeding infant
Identify stool patterns for breast-fed infants	
Discuss need to increase frequency (scheduling every 2 hours) of breast-feeding during growth spurts	
Discuss use of nutrient supplements while breast-feeding	
Discuss desirable effects of lactation on involution; relate to "afterpains"	
Discuss engorgement and its treatment and provide more guidance during this time	
Verify knowledge of return of ovulation and menses while breast-feeding.	
Discuss conception control if indicated	

Continued.

NURSING CARE OF MATERNITY CLIENTS—cont'd
Knowledge deficit (breast feeding)

Etiology	Goals	Nursing intervention	Outcome criteria
		Reinforce teaching with audiovisual aids	
		Relate factors that influence milk supply, e.g., smoking, alcohol, rest	
		Supply mother with list of community resources available for guidance, e.g., Childbirth Education Association, LaLeche League, hospital program	
		Be a source of support during process	

NURSING CARE OF MATERNITY CLIENTS
Parenting, alteration in: potential
Donna Lawrence, R.N., M.S.

Etiology	Goals	Nursing intervention	Outcome criteria
Adolescent parent(s) with unmet maturational needs	To support constructive parenting	Establish effective trust relationship with family	By hospital discharge time, mother and family will display increased comfort with newborn, as follows:
Lack of maturity of caregiver(s)		Assess and record observations of family interactions	
Lack of effective role models		Provide opportunity for parent(s) to express thought about parent role and care giving responsibilities	Demonstrate increasing bonding behaviors
Absence of extended family		Evaluate knowledge level of parent(s) relative to newborn and their capabilities and limitations.	Be able to appropriately console the newborn.
Lack of effective coping mechanisms		Assess if plans are realistic (for child care and support)	Provide for physical care needs of infant
Presence of stressors:		Identify newborn characteristics and capabilities—Brazelton assessment	
Physical			

Continued.

93

NURSING CARE OF MATERNITY CLIENTS—cont'd

Parenting, alteration in: potential

Etiology	Goals	Nursing intervention	Outcome criteria
Emotional		Provide role model for parent(s) with care giving activities and stimulation of infant	Have realistic understanding of newborn needs and abilities
Financial		Encourage contact with newborn in hospital; provide nonthreatening environment	Have determined support system within the family and environment
History of neglected childhood		Provide for comfort needs of mother before interactions	List community resources available for new parents
		Discuss newborn status with family	Express ways of balancing needs of all family members appropriately
		Provide opportunity for parent(s) to provide physical care of newborn in hospital	Express positive feelings about parenting and about infant
		Praise mother and/or father in care giver role when appropriate; offer constructive suggestions in nonthreatening manner	
		Encourage verbalization and tactile and visual stimulation of infant	

Identify cues of newborn, e.g., need to rest, need to be consoled

Evaluate attachment process, bonding behaviors, reciprocal interaction

Observe parent's behaviors and efforts to console crying baby; point out successful interventions

Determine extended family constellation to identify appropriate role models or alternate role models within family environment

Identify support systems within the family

List resources available within the community for financial, psychologic, social, and emergency support

Provide guidelines for entrance into health care system for care

Initiate social service consultation to evaluate family resources and needs

Initiate community health nursing referral

NURSING CARE OF PATIENTS WITH PSYCHIATRIC–MENTAL HEALTH PROBLEMS*†
Mild anxiety, moderate anxiety, severe anxiety, extreme anxiety (panic)

Gertrude K. McFarland, R.N., M.S.N., D.N.Sc.
and Evelyn L. Wasli, R.N., M.S.N. D.N.Sc.

Etiology	Defining characteristics	Nursing assessment
Perceived/actual failure of adaptive coping skills Perceived/actual threats to biologic integrity Perceived/actual threats to meaningful interpersonal relationships Perceived/actual threats to self-esteem	*Mild anxiety* Slight discomfort Enhanced ability to deal with problems Increased awareness and perception Increased problem-solving abilities Increased alertness Repetitive questioning Attention-seeking Belittling	1. What level of anxiety does patient manifest? Physiologic signs present? 2. Identify adaptive or maladaptive behavioral responses to anxiety in past and present

*The contents of this table reflect the ideas of the authors, Gertrude K. McFarland and Evelyn L. Wasli, and are not necessarily those of the U.S. Department of Health and Human Services, USPHS, Health Resources and Services Administration, Rockville, Md., and the National Institute of Mental Health, St. Elisabeths Hospital, Washington, D.C.

†Adapted from McFarland, G., and Wasli, E.: Psychiatric nursing. Part 2. In Brunner, L., and Suddarth, D.: The Lippincott manual of nursing practice, ed. 3, Philadelphia, 1982, J.B. Lippincott Co., pp. 905–983.

Nursing goals and interventions	Outcome criteria

A. To prevent or reduce anxiety to a level at which problem solving can be effective
 	
  1. Be an active listener
 	
  2. Engage in recreational and diversional activities aimed at reducing anxiety: group singing, volley ball, ping-pong, walking, swimming, simple concrete tasks, simple games, routine tasks, housekeeping chores, grooming, puzzles, cards, etc.
 	
  3. Develop a positive interpersonal relationship with the patient
 	
  4. Administer tranquilizers or sedative drugs as prescribed
	1. Anxiety reduced to level at which problem solving can be effective
	
	2. Patient recognizes presence of anxiety and develops insight into cause
	
	3. Patient uses adaptive coping strategies and behavioral responses

Continued.

‡Panel of expert reviewers on nursing diagnosis of anxiety: Sandra Bauer, R.N., M.S.N.; Anna Burnett, R.N.; Ellen Calhoun, R.N., M.S.N.; Zola Green, R.N., M.S.N.; Elizabeth Mandapat, R.N., A.D.; Mary Markert, R.N., M.N.; Hattie Matthews, R.N., D.P.H.; Charlotte Naschinski, R.N., M.S.; Karen Scipio-Skinner, R.N., M.S.N.; Clotilde Vidoni, R.N.C., M.S.N.—all of St. Elizabeths Hospital, NIMH, DHHS, Washington, D.C. Patricia O'Brien, R.N., M.S.N.—Washington Adventist Hospital, Takoma Park, Md. Glynn Hamilton, R.N., M.N.—Army Nurse Corps. Mary Attebury, R.N., M.S.; Edythe Lawrence, R.N., B.S.N.; Harriet Maier, R.N., B.S.N.; Janice Roy-Byrne, R.N., B.S.N.; Nancy Stinemetz, R.N., B.S.N.; Sandra Summers, R.N.—all of Psychiatric Institute, Washington, D.C.

**NURSING CARE OF PATIENTS WITH
PSYCHIATRIC–MENTAL HEALTH PROBLEMS**—cont'd
**Mild anxiety, moderate anxiety, severe anxiety,
extreme anxiety (panic)**

Etiology	Defining characteristics	Nursing assessment
Perceived/actual threats to value systems and ideals	Misunderstandings Restlessness Irritability Increased attention to problem situation Tension-relieving behaviors such as finger or foot tapping, nail biting, fidgeting, lip chewing *Moderate anxiety* Moderate discomfort Increased ability to concentrate and focus on problem situation Increased concentration on sensory data relevant to problem Increased verbalization Increased alertness Narrowing of perceptual field and selective inattention Voice tremors Change in voice pitch	3. Identify and continue to observe for stressors or threats generating anxiety 4. What behavioral/ physiologic changes indicating anxiety are present? 5. What does patient verbalize about state of discomfort? 6. What resources are available to the patient to deal with anxiety, e.g., significant others, clergy, therapy, recreational activities

Nursing goals and interventions	Outcome criteria
5. Encourage ventilation of feelings, considering readiness of patient	
6. Do not probe if patient is experiencing severe or extreme anxiety	
7. Be calm	
a. Avoid becoming anxious reciprocally	
b. Recognize anxiety in own self and develop control over one's own responses	
8. Use short, simple sentences and a calm, firm tone in speaking with a highly anxious patient	
9. Avoid requests for decision making, asking for cause of behavior, or making interpretations when patient is highly anxious	
10. Provide simple, brief, and clear information about experiences to be encountered while hospitalized; provide, clarify, or validate information as necessary	
11. Convey empathy, unconditional positive regard, and congruence	
12. Offer reassurance, including use of nonverbal behavior such as quiet physical presence and use of touch	
13. Intervene early to prevent escalation of anxiety to severe or extreme levels	

Continued.

Etiology	Defining characteristics	Nursing assessment
	Increased respiratory and heart rates	
	Increased muscle tension	
	Diaphoresis	
	Shakiness	
	Pacing	
	Frequency	
	Urgency	
	Somatic complaints	
	Sleeplessness	
	Severe anxiety	
	Dissociation of anxious feelings from self	
	Denial of existence of uncomfortable feelings	
	Reduced range of perception with focus on small or scattered detail	
	Inability to see connections between events or detail	
	Selective inattention	

Nursing goals and interventions	Outcome criteria
14. Keep highly anxious patient in a calm milieu	
a. Remove patient from stress if anxiety level is high until patient is less sensitive to situation	
b. Limit contact with other anxious patients	
15. Employ comfort measures such as warm bath and rest	
16. Convey attitude that a constructive resolution can be found	
17. Avoid anxiety-provoking situations, e.g., threats, insincerity, focus on weakness, indiscriminate use of psychiatric or medical terminology, unreasonable demands, indiscriminate use of confrontation of behavior, indifference or unconcerned attitude, blocking patient's rights or goals, judgmental attitude, impatience	
18. Mutually develop daily schedule of activities incorporating patient's preferences and strengths	
19. During short-term hospitalization offer additional support and assistance in dealing with anxiety on admission, on about the fifth day, and on notification of discharge	

Continued.

NURSING CARE OF PATIENTS WITH PSYCHIATRIC–MENTAL HEALTH PROBLEMS—cont'd
Mild anxiety, moderate anxiety, severe anxiety, extreme anxiety (panic)

Etiology	Defining characteristics	Nursing assessment
	Ineffective functioning	
	Difficult and inappropriate verbalizations	
	Inability to concentrate	
	Purposeless activity	
	Inability to learn	
	Sense of impending doom	
	Hyperventilation	
	Tachycardia	
	Frequency and urgency	
	Nausea	
	Headache	
	Dizziness	
	Sleeplessness	
	Extreme anxiety (panic)	
	Extreme discomfort	
	Immobility	
	Unrealistic perception of situation	
	Dilated pupils	

Nursing goals and interventions	Outcome criteria
20. Permit crying	
B. To help recognize presence of anxiety, develop insight into cause, and develop adaptive coping strategies and behavior responses	
1. If anxiety is at moderate level	
a. Help patient to identify anxiety by asking questions such as "Are you uncomfortable right now?" Point out your awareness of patient's discomfort by providing feedback on nonverbal behaviors that indicate anxiety	
b. Assist in discovering similarity of the immediate situation and past experiences in which similar discomfort was experienced; Ask questions such as, "Have you, in the past, ever felt like you feel right now? What was happening then to you? What did you do to feel less anxious?"	
c. Ask patient to describe what was desired, thought, or expected before becoming anxious and to discover the relationship of patient's state of anxiety to consequent adaptive or maladaptive behavior	

Continued.

Etiology	Defining characteristics	Nursing assessment
	Pallor	
	Disruption of perceptual field with distortion and enlargement of detail	
	Inability to speak	
	Unintelligible communication	
	Vomiting	
	Feeling of personality disintegration	
	Severe shakiness	
	Severe hyperactivity	
	Sleeplessness	

Nursing goals and interventions	Outcome criteria
d. Explore possible reasons for anxiety with patient; help patient to realistically clarify nature of problem	
e. Assist in developing alternative methods to reduce anxiety, in choosing solutions to problem, and in implementing solutions to problem(s)	
f. Evaluate results with patient	
1) Seek additional information and alternative action if plan was unsuccessful	
2) Encourage patient to refrain from being negatively judgmental about self	
2. Encourage new interests and hobbies and/or participation in familiar ones	
3. After anxiety is lowered and relationship with staff member is established	
a. Encourage social activities despite reluctance and fears	
b. Accompany patient to activity first few times and permit departure if patient becomes too anxious	
c. Gradually encourage attendance independent of staff support	

Continued.

Mild anxiety, moderate anxiety, severe anxiety,
extreme anxiety (panic)

Etiology	Defining characteristics	Nursing assessment

Nursing goals and interventions	Outcome criteria
4. Utilize and assist patient in choosing objective environmental interventions to deal with anxiety if patient is basically optimistic, open to experience, and flexible	
5. Assist patient in developing a more optimistic and constructive world view if patient's subjective work is deadened, closed, or distorted; Assist in reducing life-style of negative expectations	
6. Allow patient freedom to work at own level and pace in solving own problems	
7. Reduce secondary gains patient achieves from maladaptive behavioral responses	
C. To promote health and prevent severe anxiety	
1. Explore upcoming event; use role playing to help cope with anxiety-provoking encounters	
2. Teach patient	
a. That some anxiety is part of living and that enduring mild anxiety can enhance learning, problem solving, and movement toward self-actualization	

Continued.

NURSING CARE OF PATIENTS WITH PSYCHIATRIC–MENTAL HEALTH PROBLEMS—cont'd
Mild anxiety, moderate anxiety, severe anxiety, extreme anxiety (panic)

Etiology	Defining characteristics	Nursing assessment

BIBLIOGRAPHY

Books

Grosicki, J., editor: Nursing action guide, Washington, D.C., 1972, Veteran's Administration.

Kim, M. J., and Moritz, D. A., editors: Classification of nursing diagnoses, New York, 1982, McGraw-Hill Book Co.

McFarland, G., and Wasli, E.: Psychiatric nursing. In Brunner, L., and Suddarth, D.: Lippincott manual of nursing practice, Philadelphia, J. B. Lippincott Co., 1982.

Nursing goals and interventions	Outcome criteria
b. To observe what is happening, describe situation, analyze what patient expected and how it differs from the actual situation, develop alternatives to solve problem or change expectations, and validate situation with others	
c. Assertive communication skills	
d. Progressive muscular relaxation	
3. Instruct patient to reduce severe or extreme anxiety through talking to someone; walking; simple games; simple, concrete tasks; sports; or, if anxiety is extreme, by seeking professional help	

Articles

Holderby, R., and McNulty, F.: Feelings, feelings. Nurs. '79, 9(10):39–43, Oct. 1979.

Kerr, N.: Anxiety: theoretical considerations, Perspect. Psychiatr. Care 16(1):36–40, 46, Jan.-Feb. 1978.

Knowles, R.: Dealing with feelings: managing anxiety, Am. J. Nurs. 1:110–111, Jan. 1981.

Kristic, J.: Anxiety levels of hospitalized psychiatric patients throughout total hospitalization, *J. Psychiatr. Nurs.* 17(7):33–34, 37–42, July 1979.

Liebowitz, M., and Klein, D.: Case 1: assessment and treatment of phobic anxiety, J. Clin. Psychol. 40(11):486–492, Nov. 1979.

Pfeiffer, E.: Handling the distressed older patient, Geriatrics 34(2):24–25, 28–29, Feb. 1979.

NURSING CARE OF PATIENTS
WITH PSYCHIATRIC–MENTAL HEALTH PROBLEMS*†
Grieving: dysfunctional, potential dysfunctional

Gertrude K. McFarland, R.N., M.S.N., D.N.Sc.
and Evelyn L. Wasli, R.N., M.S.N., D.N.Sc.

Etiology	Defining characteristics	Nursing assessment
Perceived/actual loss of significant other	*Immediate physical symptoms of short duration*	1. What is the nature of the loss? When did it occur?
Perceived/actual loss of object	Sighing respirations	2. How did the patient perceive the loss? Special meaning or value? Significance of loss in relation to patient's perceived and real abilities to meet his own needs?
Significant change in life pattern and style	Choking sensation	
Loss of body part or function	Empty feeling in stomach, digestive upsets	
	Physical distress	
	Shortness of breath	
	Other symptoms developing shortly after loss	3. What stage of grieving and behavioral manifestations does patient currently present?
	Apathy	
	Depersonalization	
	Numbness; pain; disorganization	

*The contents of this table reflect the ideas of the authors, Gertrude K. McFarland and Evelyn L. Wasli, and are not necessarily those of the U.S. Department of Health and Human Services, USPHS, Health Resources and Services Administration, Rockville, Md., and the National Institute of Mental Health, St. Elisabeths Hospital, Washington, D.C.

Nursing goals and interventions	Outcome criteria

A. To facilitate normal grieving
 	
  1. Assist patient through denial phase
 	
    a. Help patient understand that others respond similarly when grieving a loss
 	
    b. Be genuine, honest, and realistic about loss
 	
    c. Permit visual and tactile contact with body of dead when possible
 	
    d. Use caring tone of voice
 	
  2. Assist patient through anger phase
 	
    a. Demonstrate tolerance, patience, and empathy
 	
    b. Permit open expression of feelings; do not become defensive
 	
    c. Assist patient in understanding reasons for feelings
	1. Patient resolves loss through normal grieving process
	
	2. Patient uses coping strategies and engages in constructive life-style

Continued.

†Adapted from McFarland, G., and Wasli, E.: Psychiatric nursing. Part 2. In Brunner, L., and Suddarth, D.: The Lippincott manual of nursing practice, ed. 3, Philadelphia, 1982, J.B. Lippincott Co., pp. 905–983.

**NURSING CARE OF PATIENTS WITH
PSYCHIATRIC–MENTAL HEALTH PROBLEMS—cont'd**
Grieving: dysfunctional, potential dysfunctional

Etiology	Defining characteristics	Nursing assessment
	High degree of organization followed by collapse, shock, disbelief, hyperactivity, hypersomnolence, bewilderment, confusion, restlessness, lack of strength, aimless activity, meaninglessness of daily routine, withdrawal, immobile behavior	4. Describe patient's behavior between actual occurrence of loss and present
		5. How has patient coped with loss in the past? What strengths were demonstrated in coping with loss?
	Stages of functional grieving	
	Denial—avoids acceptance of loss, thereby developing a buffer against reality	6. Determine whether patient is at high risk for dysfunctional grieving; examples are those with
	1. Acts as if deceased is still present or loss has not occurred; searching behavior	a. Poor relationship with person before death
		b. Social isolation or poor social network

Nursing goals and interventions	Outcome criteria
d. If patient has difficulty in expressing anger, place with patients who can express feelings openly	
e. Reassure patient that feelings of guilt are part of the normal grieving process; assist in working through feelings of guilt	
f. Encourage patient to work out conflicting aspect of relationship with deceased; work through any ambivalence	
3. Assist patient through bargaining phase	
a. Permit patient's need to talk and reminisce about loss through active listening	
b. Permit expression of feelings and thoughts. Gently point out reality	
4. Assist through realization of loss phase	
a. Be physically present; offer support and enhance self-esteem	
b. Offer acceptance and unconditional positive regard	
c. Correct misinformation about cause of loss	

Continued.

NURSING CARE OF PATIENTS WITH PSYCHIATRIC–MENTAL HEALTH PROBLEMS—cont'd
Grieving: dysfunctional, potential dysfunctional

Etiology	Defining characteristics	Nursing assessment
	2. Other characteristics can include disinterest in environment, withdrawal, immobility, decreased responsiveness, occurrence of fantasies about loss	c. History of multiple past losses and use of maladaptive coping strategies
	3. Begins to mobilize other coping strategies	d. Presentation of a brave, stoic front
	Anger—channeled toward lost object or person, toward self, or displaced toward other object or person	7. What is the nature of the social network present?
	1. Questions reasons for happening: "Why did this happen to me?"	8. Assess degree of depression; observe for suicidal tendencies
	2. Experiences guilt along with self-criticism and self-punishing behavior	9. What are significant others' reaction to patient's response to loss?
	3. May place blame on health professionals or may misinterpret what is said by them	

Nursing goals and interventions	Outcome criteria
d. Reinforce past and present strengths in dealing with difficulty	
e. Through sympathetic understanding show that crying is acceptable	
f. Encourage support for patient from family members and friends	
g. Observe for and monitor depression	
h. Facilitate review of positive and negative aspects of lost person, object, or life pattern	
i. Clarify and offer missing factual information	
j. Use touch to offer support	
5. Assist through acceptance phase	
a. Explore nature of problems encountered that are linked to loss	
b. Raise questions regarding next steps in coping	
c. Assist analysis of adaptive coping strategies	
d. Assist or coordinate resources to develop new skills, to make readjustments in life-style, and to make new emotional investments	

Continued.

Grieving: dysfunctional, potential dysfunctional

Etiology	Defining characteristics	Nursing assessment
	4. Other characteristics can include irritability, fear, lack of sleep	
	Bargaining—last attempt to postpone realization of loss, which may include bargaining with a deity	
	1. Seeks magical cures	
	2. Attempts to negotiate for change in reality	
	3. Preoccupied with image of deceased	
	Realization of loss—full awareness of loss, including meaning and value of person or object to self, awareness of lost or changed roles, realization of new responsibilities and roles	
	1. Preoccupation with loss	

Nursing goals and interventions	Outcome criteria
e. Support patient who is trying out new coping strategies	
6. Do not suppress symptoms of grieving with drugs; suggest use of willpower or other verbal interventions	
7. Answer questions directly and tactfully	
8. Orient patient to new aspects of environment in a simple and clear way	
9. Foster environment in which loss can be placed in spiritual context by engaging patient in religious and spiritual rituals and practices as desired	
10. Be cognizant of the possibility of different stages of grieving occurring among family members; help patient and family members communicate with each other	
11. Offer extensive support and guidance in performing activities of living during bewilderment experienced immediately after loss	
12. Demonstrate caring and concern, especially immediately after the loss	

Continued.

**NURSING CARE OF PATIENTS WITH
PSYCHIATRIC–MENTAL HEALTH PROBLEMS—cont'd**
Grieving: dysfunctional, potential dysfunctional

Etiology	Defining characteristics	Nursing assessment
	2. Can include symptoms of depressive behavior, such as despair, crying, inertia, withdrawal, emptiness, helplessness, hopelessness, loneliness	
	Acceptance and reintegration—problem-solving behavior initiated relative to loss and concomitant problems and change	
	1. Renewal of energy in living	
	2. Development of new, emotional investments	
	3. Ability to realistically remember both positive and negative aspects of the lost person, object, or life pattern	
	4. Restructuring and reordering of life	

Nursing goals and interventions	Outcome criteria
13. Encourage patient to seek help and not be "too proud"	
14. Use role play as a way to help work through feelings	
15. Do not abandon patient who is experiencing loss	
16. Provide anticipatory guidance and support anticipatory grieving	
B. To resolve dysfunctional grieving	
1. Apply interventions outlined for normal grieving	
2. Assist patient in getting through phase in which patient is stuck	
a. Assess present stage of grieving and the current objects or facts that patient still links to the loss	
b. Use graded flooding approach	
1) Present patient with increasing significant facts about or objects linked to loss	
2) Rework feelings generated	
3) Use role play to work through feelings and preoccupations	
4) Apply principles of behavior modification, such as rewards for more adaptive behavior	

Continued.

**NURSING CARE OF PATIENTS WITH
PSYCHIATRIC–MENTAL HEALTH PROBLEMS**—cont'd
Grieving: dysfunctional, potential dysfunctional

Etiology	Defining characteristics	Nursing assessment
	Characteristics of dysfunctional grieving	
	Excessive emotional reaction	
	Arrested or excessive time in any phase of grieving	
	Prolonged excessive denial of loss	
	Prolonged depression	

Nursing goals and interventions	Outcome criteria
3. Offer extra assistance in process or grieving to those at high risk for dysfunctional grieving. Examples are	
a. Those who had a traumatic, difficult relationship with person who is now deceased	
b. Those who are socially isolated or who have a poorly developed social network	
c. Those who present cheerful, brave, and stoic behavior	
d. Those who have a history of multiple past losses and have used maladaptive coping strategies	
e. Those who perceive their social network as nonsupportive	
f. Those with very traumatic circumstances surrounding death of spouse—anger or guilt-provoking death, unexpected or untimely death	
g. Those with concurrent life crises	
C. To promote health and prevent dysfunctional grieving	
1. Teach patient to	
a. Define potential life changes and problems predicted from the loss	

Continued.

NURSING CARE OF PATIENTS WITH
PSYCHIATRIC–MENTAL HEALTH PROBLEMS—cont'd
Grieving: dysfunctional, potential dysfunctional

Etiology	Defining characteristics	Nursing assessment

BIBLIOGRAPHY

Books

Brown, M., and Hess, P.: Nursing and the concept of loss, New York, 1980, John Wiley & Sons, Inc.

Caplan, G.: Principles of preventive psychiatry, New York, 1964, Basic Books, Inc., Publishers.

Doyle, P.: Grief counseling and sudden death, Springfield, 1980, Charles C Thomas, Publisher.

Feifel, H.: New meanings of death, New York, 1977, McGraw-Hill Book Co.

Glaser, B., and Strauss, A.: Awareness of dying, Chicago, 1965, Aldine Publishing Co.

Nursing goals and interventions	Outcome criteria
b. Develop alternative potential strategies to deal with problems	
c. Map out possible consequences of each strategy	
d. Determine priorities of strategies in terms of usefulness for potential problem resolution	
2. Help patient to seek assistance with expected or impending loss	
3. Teach patient to openly discuss and express feelings about expected and impending loss	
4. Support patient in seeking psychologic support from clergy, significant other, or mental health professional during bereavement to reduce potential for dysfunctional grieving	

Glaser, B., and Strauss, A.: Time for dying, Chicago, 1968, Aldine Publishing Co.

Glick, I., Weiss, R., and Parkes, C.: The first year of bereavement, New York, 1974, John Wiley & Sons, Inc.

Kubler-Ross, E.: On death and dying, New York, 1969, Macmillan Publishing Co.

Lindemann, E.: Beyond grief, studies in crisis intervention, New York, 1979, Jason Aronson, Inc.

McFarland, G., and Wasli, E.: Psychiatric nursing. In Brunner, L., and Suddarth, D.: Lippincott manual of nursing practice, Philadelphia, 1982, J. B. Lippincott Co.

Simos, B.: A time to grieve, New York, 1979, Family Service Association of America.

Simpson, M.: Dying, death, and grief, New York, 1979, Plenum Press.

Werner-Beland, J., and Agee, J.: Grief responses to long-term illness and disability, Reston, Va., 1980, Reston Publishing Co.

Articles

Asbury, B., Barton, D., Barton, L, et al.: What can you give for grief? Care, Patient care 13:100–102, 104, 108–110, 115–116, 121–122, 127–128, 131–132, March 1979.

Blanchard, C., Blanchard, E., and Becker, J.: The young widow: depressive symptomatology throughout the grief process, Psychiatry 39:394–399, Nov. 1976.

Breu, C., and Dracup, K.: Helping the spouses of critical patients, Am. J. Nurs. 78:50–53, Jan. 1978.

Clayton, P., Halikas, J., Maurice, W., et al.: Anticipatory grief and widowhood, Brit. J. Psychiatr. 122:47–51, Jan. 1973.

Coles, P.: Breaking the grief barrier, Nurs. Mirror 148:34–35, May 1979.

Courtemanche, J.: Death in emergency, Can. Nurse 74:24–26, Nov. 1978.

Dracup, K., and Breu, C.: Using nursing research findings to meet the needs of grieving spouses, Nurs. Res. 27:212–216, July-Aug. 1978.

Engel, G.: Grief and grieving, Am. J. Nurs. 64:93–98, Sept. 1964.

Freihofer, P., and Felton, G.: Nursing behaviors in bereavement: an exploratory study, Nurs. Res. 25:332–337, Sept.-Oct. 1976.

Greenblatt, M.: The grieving spouse, Am. J. Psychiatry 135:43–47, Jan. 1978.

Hodgkinson, P.: Treating abnormal grief in the bereaved, Nurs. Times 76:126–128, Jan. 1980.

Horowitz, M., Wilner, N., Marmar, C., et al.: Pathological grief and the activation of latent self-images, Am. J. Psychiatry 137:1157–1162, Oct. 1980.

Jackson, E.: Wisely managing our grief: a pastoral viewpoint, Death Education 3:143–155, Summer 1979.

Lamperelli, P., and Smith, J.: The grieving process of adoption: an application of principles and techniques, J. Psychiatric Nurs. 17:24–29, Oct. 1979.

Lindemann, E.: Symptomatology and management of acute grief, Am. J. Psychiatry 101:141–148, 1944.

McCawley, A.: Help patients cope with grief, Consultant, 17:64–67, Nov. 1977.

Pett, D.: Grief in hospital, Nurs. Times, 75:709–712, April 1979.

Raphael, B.: Preventive intervention with the recently bereaved, Arch. Gen. Psychiatry 34:1450–1454, Dec. 1977.

Schlosser, S.: The emergency c-section patient. Why she needs help. . . what you can do, RN, 41: 52–57, Sept. 1978.

Schmale, A.: Reactions to illness; convalescence and grieving, Psychiatr. Clin. North Am. 2:321–330, Aug. 1979.

Schultz, C.: The dynamics of grief, J. Emergency Nurs. 5:26–30, Sept.-Oct. 1979.

Stoller, E.: Effect of experience on nurses' responses to dying and death in the hospital setting, Nurs. Res. 29:35–38, Jan.-Feb. 1980.

Thompson, D.: Thoughts on bereavement, Nurs. Times 73:1334–1335, Aug. 1977.

Vachon, M.: Grief and bereavement following the death of a spouse, Can. Psychiatr. Assoc. J. 21:25–43, Feb. 1976.

Weingourt, R.: Battered women: the grieving process, J. Psychiatr. Nurs. 17:40–47, April 1979.

NURSING CARE OF PATIENTS WITH RENAL TRANSPLANTS
Nutrition, alteration in: more than requirements
Lucy Feild, R.N., M.S.N.

Etiology	Goals	Nursing intervention	Outcome criteria
A. Steroid-induced increase in appetite	Restoration and maintenance of optimal nutritional level	Assess patient's knowledge base regarding balanced nutritional intake	Patient will achieve and maintain ideal and/or desired weight
		Assess pre-illness eating patterns, food preferences; assess patient-assigned values regarding eating, food, personal appearance	
		Assist patient to identify desired weight *before* transplant; discuss this in relation to ideal weight	
		Encourage patient to institute a low-fat, low-salt, high-protein diet, depending on renal function and physician's orders, if renal function has returned to normal	
		Encourage patient to eat moderate-sized portions, establish a regular meal pattern, and avoid snacking,	

	particularly in the immediate post-transplant period when appetite is most enhanced	Same as in A
	Assist patient to identify strategies to prevent excess weight gain	
	Monitor posttransplant nutrition intake and daily weights	
	Refer to dietician as indicated for diet teaching, meal planning, and obesity control	
B. Psychosocial factors Anxiety Depression Pre-illness eating patterns Excess intake of calories in response to stress Self-concept of heavier than ideal weight	Recognize that weight gain or obesity may be symptomatic of another problem; assess patient concerns, coping patterns, and self-concept and proceed accordingly if another diagnosis exists	

NURSING CARE OF PATIENTS WITH RENAL TRANSPLANTS
Self-concept, disturbance in: body image
Lucy Feild, R.N., M.S.N.

Etiology	Goals	Nursing intervention	Outcome criteria

	Restoration and maintenance of satisfaction with body image	*General interventions*
		1. Monitor for signs and symptoms: verbal or nonverbal response to actual or perceived change in body image
		
		  a. Avoidance and/or neglect of body part
		
		  b. Hiding or overexposing affected body part
		
		  c. Change in socialization patterns
		
		  d. Verbalized fear of rejection or negative reaction by others
		
		  e. Verbalized negative feelings about body
		
		  f. Verbalized feelings of loss and associated emotional responses
			The patient will
			
			Provide optimum care to body parts
			
			Report satisfaction and comfort with social interaction patterns
			
			Verbalize feelings of self-acceptance
			
			State that coping behaviors for dealing with perceived changes are successful

Continued.

g. Depersonalization of affected body part

h. Preoccupation with perceived change or loss

i. Extension of body boundary to incorporate environmental objects (e.g., dialysis machine)

2. Encourage verbalization of feelings, perceptions; help patient identify perceived meaning of changes

3. Convey attitude of understanding, openness, and acceptance, with focus on value of patient as a person

4. Assist patient to maintain optimum hygiene and grooming

5. Help patient identify, appreciate, and maximize strengths and assets

6. Consult with other health care team members as indicated

NURSING CARE OF PATIENTS WITH RENAL TRANSPLANTS—cont'd

Self-concept, disturbance in: body image

Etiology	Goals	Nursing intervention	Outcome criteria
A. Physical changes secondary to uremia		1. Help patient recognize that patients' negative reactions to changes in appearance are normal and expected	
Skin color changes caused by urochrome deposition		2. Help patient, when ready to participate in and/or assume responsibility for care of negatively perceived body parts	
Dry hair with potential alopecia resulting from decreased sebaceous gland oil production and metabolic imbalances		3. Help patient identify ways to minimize negatively perceived aspects of appearance (e.g., use of clothing, makeup, hairstyles, etc.)	
Thin, brittle, brown-pigmented nails resulting from metabolic imbalances		4. Help patient anticipate possible reactions of others and to formulate plans for coping with these reactions	

Continued.

Decreased or absent urine output	
Impaired sexual function	
B. Vascular access	See interventions for A. Physical changes related to uremia
C. Attachment to dialysis machine	1. Reinforce reality that patient is different from machine
	2. Promote maintenance of self-esteem through provision of privacy, respect, etc.
	3. Encourage patient to view the machine as a useful piece of equipment which can be appreciated and disliked simultaneously
D. Physical changes related to transplantation	

NURSING CARE OF PATIENTS WITH RENAL TRANSPLANTS—cont'd
Self-concept, disturbance in: body image

Etiology	Goals	Nursing intervention	Outcome criteria
1. Psychologic incorporation of another person's kidney into own body image		1. Encourage patient to discuss feelings and concerns 2. Recognize the normalcy of process of integrating kidney into the body image, which occurs over about 1 year 3. Reinforce the recipient's lack of responsibility for cadaver donor's death 4. Reinforce uniqueness of both donor and recipient	

2. Steroid effects	5. Clarify reality as indicated
	6. If significant manifestations persist past 1 year in the presence of stable, adequate renal function, refer patient for counseling
	1. See general interventions
	2. See interventions for A. Physical changes related to uremia
3. Resolution of uremic appearance	See general interventions
4. Resumption of urination	See general interventions

NOTES

NOTES

NOTES

NOTES

NOTES

NOTES

NOTES

NOTES

NOTES

NOTES

NOTES

NOTES

NOTES

NOTES

NOTES

NOTES

NOTES